CHARLES de KUNFFY

A RIDER'S

SURVIVAL *FROM* TYRANNY

To Pam,
for more memories of
Budapest,
Charles de Kunffy
Feb. 14, 2014

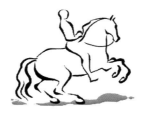

A RIDER'S

SURVIVAL FROM TYRANNY

by CHARLES de KUNFFY

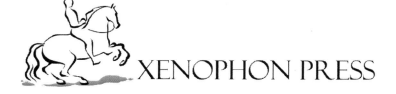

XENOPHON PRESS

Published by Xenophon Press LLC, 7518 Bayside Road, Franktown, Virginia 23354-2106, U.S.A.

Edited by Richard and Frances Williams

ISBN-10: 0933316283

ISBN-13: 978-0-933316-28-7

Front Cover: Award Ceremony for the Three Day Event April 1-4, 1956, Kossuth Academy, Budapest with high ranking military and governmental officials awarding the author on *Kormend.* Inside

Cover: The Kunffy Coat of Arms granted by the Habsburg Emperor Charles VI, rendered by E. Krahl.

Cover design by Naia Poyer.

Books written by Charles de Kunffy:
Creative Horsemanship 1975, 1984
Dressage Questions Answered 1980 1984
Training Strategies for Dressage Riders 1994, 2003
The Athletic Development of the Dressage Horse 1992
The Ethics and Passions of Dressage, 1993, 2013
Dressage Principles Illuminated 2002
A Rider's Survival from Tyranny 2012

TABLE OF CONTENTS

XENOPHON PRESS LIBRARY

30 Years with Master Nuno Oliveira, Michel Henriquet 2011
A Rider's Survival From Tyranny, Charles de Kunffy 2012
Another Horsemanship, Jean-Claude Racinet 1994
Art of the Lusitano, Pedro Yglesias de Oliveira 2012
Baucher and His School, General Decarpentry 2011
Dressage in the French Tradition, Dom Diogo de Bragança 2011
École de Cavalerie Part II , François Robichon de la Guérinière 1992
François Baucher:The Man and His Method, Hilda Nelson 2013
*From the Real Picaria of the 18th Century to the Portuguese School of
        Equestrian Art*, Yglesias de Oliveira and da Costa 2012
Healing Hands, Dominique Giniaux, DVM 1998
Methodical Dressage of the Riding Horse and *Dressage of the Outdoor
        Horse*, Faverot de Kerbrech 2010
Racinet Explains Baucher, Jean-Claude Racinet 1997
The Écuyères of the Nineteenth Century in the Circus,
        Hilda Nelson 2001
The Ethics and Passions of Dressage, Expanded Edition
        Charles de Kunffy 2013
The Gymnasium of the Horse, Gustav Steinbrecht 2011
The Handbook of Jumping Essentials, François Lemaire de
        Ruffieu 1997
The Legacy of Master Nuno Oliveira, Stephanie Millham 2013
The Maneige Royal, Antoine de Pluvinel 2010
The Spanish Riding School in Vienna and Piaffe and Passage,
        General Decarpentry 2013
The Wisdom of Master Nuno Oliveira, Antoine de Coux 2012
Total Horsemanship, Jean-Claude Racinet 1999
What the Horses have Told me, Dominique Giniaux, DVM 1996

Available at www.XenophonPress.com

ACKNOWLEDGMENTS

I am greatly indebted to the friends who volunteered to read this manuscript intending to critique it. My stories are clear to me because I was the one telling them. However, they may not be well-told if my readers cannot understand them clearly. Therefore, those who spent time and energy alerting me to needs for improvement were, to me, of great value.

I burdened my friend, Mrs. Susanne Hassler, an outstanding equestrian, by my request. Mr. Matthew Kimball, a Silicon Valley entrepreneur goaded me to write on. He red-penned the manuscript giving me additional days of silent work. My riding student and my muse, Ms. Cynthia Riley, Esquire from Santa Ynez Valley, California gave me inspiration, courage and enthusiasm to write my guarded memories. My good friend, Richard Rubinstein flooded me with ideas for improvement and demanded that I write more.

Lastly, I wish to thank my publisher, Xenophon Press for giving me the idea to write this book, and for editing, compiling and producing my memoir. Without their substantial help this project would not have been realized.

FOREWORD

These are my memories of a few years that my mother described charitably by saying "Unfortunately we live in historically interesting times." The beginning and the ending were fabulous and as Niccolo Macchiavelli advised, *"Il guarda al fine."* (Pay attention to how it ends) The years I chronicle here tested my ability to survive. I made it through these times with the help of horses and the like-minded people that loved them.

These are remembrances and they are colored by my emotions. They chronicle events the way I now remember them. These recollections are limited to a selection of those associated with my equestrian life. The truth is always more than a collection of facts.

I altered some names to protect people. This is not a documentary. I am determined to remain discreet and refuse to become a traitor.

IT HAPPENED ON NOVEMBER 6, 1956

Two days after the November fourth attack on Budapest by the newly arrived Soviet divisions, we lived under martial law and had to observe strict curfew regulations. There was a general strike. The nation refused to work for Soviet masters and Hungarians were determined to break the back of communist rule, by now with pathetic and desperate means such as striking. I was no strikebreaker but sharply at 6 a.m., when the curfew was ended, I left our apartment to go to ride my horses. Animals know nothing about national strikes and need to be both fed and exercised. I had six horses in training waiting for me and I set out on the still, dark avenues toward the riding academy.

At this stage of the Soviet occupation we were aware of sharp shooters sighting us and shooting without the slightest provocation. I always felt as if I was being viewed through the cross hairs of weapons by merciless eyes. I adopted logical life-saving strategies. One such idea was that one should not reach for a handkerchief in one's pocket, because a sniper might misinterpret that motion as reaching for a weapon. I carried my white handkerchief, in fact, in my hand, not only because my nose was running in the chilly morning, but also to make it available for lifting it up to wave the "I surrender" signal to the soldiers of communism.

With my usual outsized steps, I was striding fast to fight the cold, fear and hazards. Naively, we thought that by moving fast, bullets would not find us, thinking we would have passed the point to which the soldier aimed. Besides, my trip would be a long one since I had to walk the full length of Kossuth Avenue, continue on Rakoczi Avenue, skirt edge of the Keleti Rail Terminal and finally enter the relative safety of the riding academy.

I was walking alone on the utterly deserted avenue, thinking that all the hidden sharp shooters were behind curtains in high windows, or rooftops, or behind columns and in darkened doorways from all of which they were concentrating their aims on me. The commanders demanded "socialistic diligence" and "patriotic fervor" from their soldiers who in turn were hoping for suspicious behavior, so that they could shoot for merit and earn praise for their heroic accuracies.

Soon after I crossed the deserted Lesser Ring Boulevard and strode on to Rakoczi Avenue, I was nearing the Urania Movie Theater, looming large on the opposite side of the street. There, walking frighteningly synchronized with my steps, in rhythm with my strides, was a patrolling Soviet soldier. Suddenly, unexpectedly, from a side street, a small child appeared unaccompanied and walked jauntily toward the Soviet soldier. He was a little boy, heavily clad in oversized, rumpled, rag-tag shabby clothing. He appeared to have been as young as six years old or maybe an emaciated nine-year-old. There he was, with his brave strides approaching the Soviet patrol and when arriving at the Urania Movie Theater, he took a white sheet of paper out of his soiled jacket – very likely a revolutionary leaflet in Hungarian – and proceeded to tape it onto the glass door of the theater. As he was diligently struggling with his little hands to make the paper stick to the door, the Soviet soldier stepped closer and shot him in the head from behind.

They were both in full view to me as I was still on approach to the Urania. Realizing that I was the only witness to this act of heartless barbarism I almost threw up in my panic, fearing for my miserable life. Witnesses were routinely "eliminated" even for trivia. My neck stiffened and locked into a position from which I could not move it to turn my head, yet I could still see from a distance that the soldier now pointed the barrel of his submachine gun on to me. My riding pants were suddenly soaked and my left boot filled with warm urine as I involuntarily wetted myself, amazingly while walking. My strides got stiffer as it took the greatest concentration to keep my strides steady, and my direction straight because I felt near faint and worried about losing direction. As if drunk, I worried about losing control of how I walked and frightened myself when I thought of staggering. Near mindless with sorrow and feeling dazed, I had to pretend that I was perfectly well and that I did not notice anything unusual. Pretending ignorance was always a lifesaver in a tyranny, for noticing anything could easily have given me the death sentence. I was the only witness, not that it mattered. In a war everyone has a death sentence on his head, only some are not executed because of a lack of time or slothfulness of effort.

As if commanded by an outside force, I obeyed blindly the wisdom of pretending not to have noticed anything, or worse, seeing something significant, or Heaven forbid, witnessing something tragic. It was well known that communists, whose lies would not survive as easily, if contested by witnessed facts, always shot inconvenient witnesses. Soviet communist party members said that being a translator to Stalin was a death sentence. Hearing the words of the "great father" made translators privy to "state secrets" and they were eventually killed to prevent them from revealing these "secrets."

The little boy collapsed in a heap, soundlessly, without so much as a struggle or a yelp. He became a little grey heap of rags hiding a heroic, brave child, fallen when confronting the unfathomable. And I kept walking with my posture erect, neck locked, never turning to look, and convinced that I would be taken out next.

By the time I reached the National Theater, I reasoned that I would be out of range of the soldier's shot. My neck unlocked but I did not turn to look, for turning one's head would raise the suspicions of other sharp shooters that were hidden behind curtained windows , on rooftops and behind columns. And so it happened, that I did not get shot, but I had to watch someone else die. I reached my horses; riding them helped me live that day. I could not tell what I saw. Even now I can only write it to avoid sobbing.

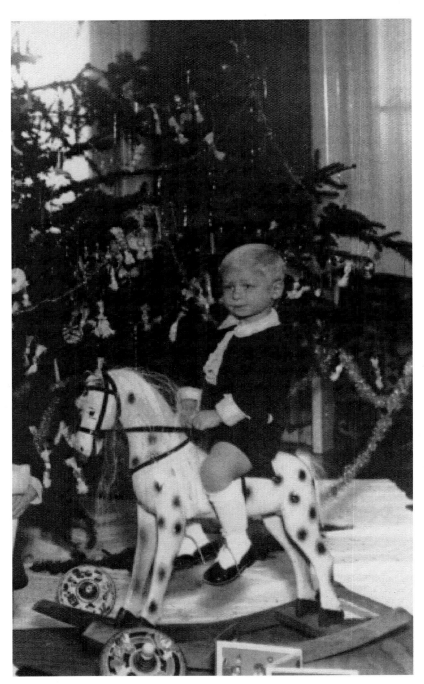

**The author, three years young,
starting his riding career early.**

CHAPTER 1

THERE WERE NO CLOUDS IN MY HEAVEN

Things were not always as tragic as on that November day. I witnessed many more horrendous events. I consider them essential parts of my privileged life. Culturally, I have lived the equivalent of two centuries. I was born into a society that was the lingering survival of "La Belle Epoch," representing the pinnacle of Western Civilization. Soon it would be replaced in Europe by the barbaric thugs that imposed totalitarian dictatorships. Yet, I survived to live the glories of the twenty-first century at its cutting-edge best in the United States.

The beginning of my life was pure enchantment. Once upon a time, my parents and I lived in a castle that was our family home. It had 45 rooms and sat in the midst of a 48-acre park in the informal "English style" and of such great beauty that foreign dignitaries desired invitations to visit. The household staff was uniformed and served in white gloves. They worshipped my parents and flooded me with sweet affection. I had a perfect governess. She was Austrian, tranquil, quiet, patient and attentive. She "abandoned me," as I used to tease her, when I was fourteen. Her name was Berta Schmalding but the whole world knew her by my nickname for her, Beci.

The castle and a large part of the estate it commanded were in my name. That was determined by procedures for appropriate inheritance. My parents were, of course, its custodians until I would reach maturity. By that time, however, the communists confiscated my property and we were exiled from the county in which we lived.

Our castle did not correspond to the images of a defense fortification. I digress to explain that in Hungary the term for a residence such as was mine was *kastely*. In German the same general concept was assigned the term *schloss*, in French, *château* and in English, castle. These expressions were not merely references to buildings of a certain size, elegant architecture and

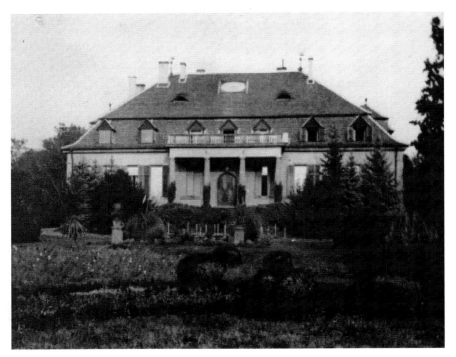

**The western façade of the 'castle'
with the colonnaded carriage entrance**

splendor. The word, *castle*, originally could refer to an ancient defense structure. However, in time it became vernacular to include more recently built palaces, mansions, and manor houses or elaborate villas. Size and architecture influenced, but were not the determining factors in how they were labeled.

The most important attribute of a castle was that it conveyed more than a large, elegant, even opulent residence. On post cards depicting such residences the words kastely, schloss, chateau and castle all appeared. It was the life conducted in them that was the common denominator in defining a castle.

Castles, including the one in which I lived until I was fourteen, were not only great houses, but were also repositories of culture, homes to patronage, centers of charities, examples of traditional duties for caring for others and performing duties toward employees and the nation. Eminent artists, scientists, architects, scholars and statesmen visited castles. They were the places where aristocrats vied to produce the best concerts,

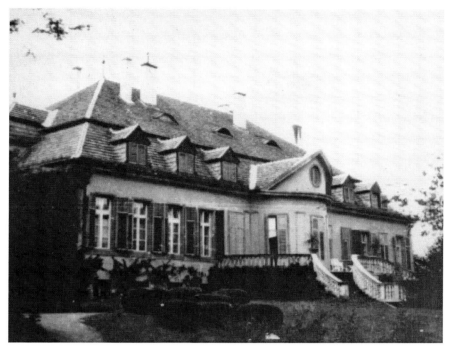

The eastern façade with the grand terrace

create the finest gardens, erect monuments to cultural tradition, celebrate the spirits of a particular age, and maintain a temple to the arts they collected. The residents of castles were respected, admired even adored as conscientious and duty-bound producers of food, fuel and the necessities of life. The traditional obligations of the aristocracy also included the provision of justice and the defense of the nation. The aristocracy was respected, because they earned their titles and privileges by serving well, conscientiously and to the benefit of others in the nation. Aristocrats were raised to their privileged positions by having rendered special services to the nation. On the whole, they were decent, caring, duty-bound and honorable.

My large family, members of them titled, lived in castles. Mine was one of the smaller, more modest ones, built in 1901 by my grandparents who adored the quiet simplicity of country life. The exotic and magnificent park was completed in 1911.

Our castle was grand, yet cozy. It seemed enormous and imposing at times while minutes later it might feel intimate and

11

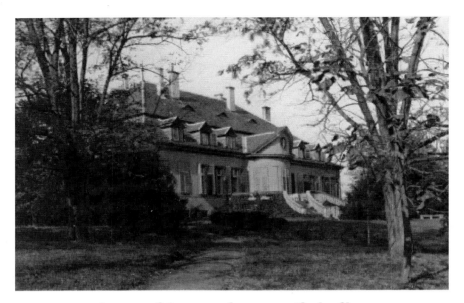

Approaching on a long, gentle incline

comforting. As most castles, mine was primarily a beautifully comfortable home, yet elegant for hosting grand receptions. It reclined on a modest hill in softly undulating terrain that was transformed into the most beautiful park I had ever seen. In centuries past, these same lands were pastures. On them stood six gigantic Dutch Elm trees, under which cattle rested in the shade. These survivors were estimated to have lived there for seven hundred years. The foremost garden architect of Victorian England designed the park as a "Garden of Eden" for my Anglophile grandparents. Trees, shrubs and flowers were imported from all continents, except Antarctica, to join the great elms and combined into a visual triumph that never ceased to amaze, delight and enchant those fortunate occupants. State guests and eminent foreign travelers visited the park on the recommendation of the Ministry of Agriculture.

My parents were legendary for their hospitality. When the grand salon of the castle was populated with a large number of eminent guests, the governess trotted me out for everyone's inspection. Splendidly attired in a midnight blue velvet suit with lace collar and striding in patent leather shoes, I was carrying myself bolt upright. I had better manners then than now, as I

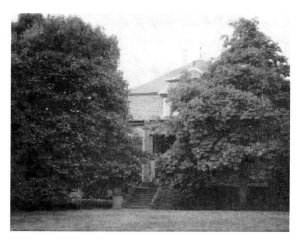

My bedroom is behind the large maple on the left.

have regrettably out-grown them for lack of practice. But when I was a little child, I could go from eminent guest to more eminent guests, bow to the appropriate level of depth, kiss a lady's hand or a bishop's ring effortlessly, greet each guest properly and respond to small conversations without fluster.

There would be dukes, bishops, famous professors, opera divas, movie stars, exotic hunters, Olympic athletes, a sprinkling of Italian counts, some British academicians, and even some fab-

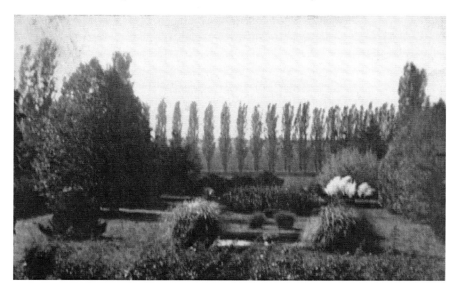

**The poplar avenue bearing my name
was the grand approach to the park.
The tranquil fountain is visible in the center.**

13

ulously beautiful relatives. Often conversation was conducted in four different languages in the same room. Between the age of 3 and 5, I was frequently asked by these guests, "What do you want to be when you grow up?" Without hesitation and with great earnestness and sincerity I replied, "I will be a pig herd." I noticed some suppressed amusement pass over the faces of the inquiring guests followed by the question, "But why be a pig herd?" And I reassured them of the obvious reasons. "Because I want to have those spotted herding dogs and lean on my staff,

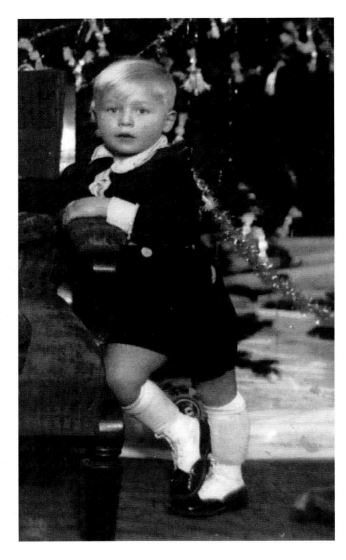

Ready for inspection by the guests.

14

watching them herd the pigs." Well, that seemed to have satisfied the curiosity of any of those adults.

By the time I was about five, I made a career change decision. From then on, the eminent guests would hear my reply: "I will be a coachman and drive carriages." The expected follow-up question was, "But why?" I answered, "Because I like the uniforms and I love to watch the horses when they are swiftly trotting." Well, that was also satisfactory but my father ruined it for me by laughing loudly and saying, "I will hire you." I did not want that at all.

With respect to the socioeconomic picture, there was a long-standing tradition of interdependence of people from different levels of society. We owned three villages and my father employed all of the inhabitants who wished to work. The villagers adored my parents and none would leave. The ideal of all great estates was self-sufficiency. First of all, estates were managed to provide goods, livelihood and wellbeing to the local peasantry. Surpluses and special crops were marketed and reached the capital daily and were also shipped to foreign countries. Everyone knew their place and was content, well aware of their value. Loyalty and trust prevailed. The success of my parents' enterprises were appreciated, enjoyed, and praised by the laborers. The villagers exhibited great pride in the estate's successes and were known to boast of them. These successes came from hard labor.

One of the most sought after advancement in the life of a villager was to work at the castle and to be admitted to the household staff. Any position of personal service filled the employed with pride and elevated them to a higher class of service and life with prospects for a much better marriage. They acquired skills, manners, education, poise and charm by living and serving in a great house.

His societal peers mockingly called my father "The socialist landlord." He earned this description because he loved all his employees and all the villagers and treated them with unique generosity. He built for the villagers an Olympic size swimming pool and maintained it impeccably. To my knowledge, nowhere else in Hungary was an estate with a resort-sized swimming

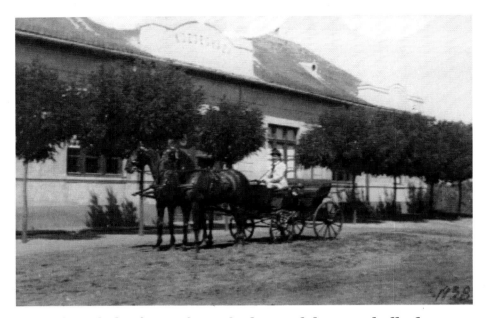

One of my father's carriages in front of the townhall of our village. The two mares were *Koszeg* and *Hernad,* a perfectly matched pair of red bays that were full sisters born one year apart. The driver in his summer uniform and elegant posture.

pool provided only for the peasantry. Father also designated a carriage and driver for anyone to use at any time if in need of visiting doctors, dentists or any other medical attendant. He provided all villagers with fuel for cooking and heating and all the salt needed for cooking and preserving food.

Most remarkably my father told the villagers that if any of their children were to matriculate from high school, he would finance their entire university education. Ironically, one of the beneficiaries of father's generous offer for a university education was a young man that finished law school and became a dreaded prosecutor later, under the communist regime.

Mutual affection, impeccable loyalty, honesty and respect were simply undisputed in our villages. The proof of it is as simple to document as my being here to write about it in California, because any person in our service could have facilitated our death. We did not take flight from the approaching Soviet

16

My mother's carriage on the avenue to the park, mother hidden under the parasol. The driver wears the white summer uniform and hard hat decorated with a white crane feather. The horse on the right was *Primadonna* imported from Italy, and the one on the left was *Dongo*.

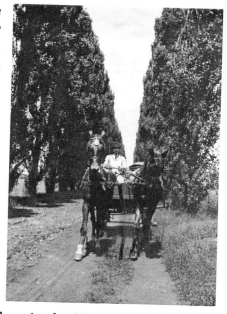

Red Army to seek American asylum in the West. Instead we remained at our estate with the naïve belief that we could protect the peasantry. Any one of three thousand peasants could have sent us to our death by false accusations. They could have informed on us and caused our demise a thousand times, but they never did.

My earliest memories included horses. We owned racehorses, draft horses, riding horses, cart horses, carriage horses, and, unfortunately, even ponies. During my childhood in the countryside, daily transportation was by horse drawn carriages. There were elegant Landaus, fabulous Victorias and practical Esterhazy Sand carriages, pulled by two or four in hand, depending on the rank of the occasion for elegance and gala. If a member of the high clergy, a Member of Parliament or a member of the aristocracy were to be collected at the railway station, a carriage pulled by "four-in-hand" was merited, opulently harnessed with traditional Hungarian leather latticework pulling a royal blue and black Landau carriage.

When "I was good," and I thought that I always was even if the opinion of the governess often differed, I merited the derogatory "privilege" of sitting to the left of the elegantly uniformed coachman on the driver's seat. I was, of course, observing the trotting mares, imagining that I drove them. I knew every one of them by name. My parents would test me, asking, "Which mares are in harness today?"

I knew and told their names.

"How do you know them by name?"

I answered with the obvious, "They are all different, you know."

There was a pony carriage with its own driver at my disposal. I regretted using them. They bored me. Even when trotting "full out," they progressed modestly. I preferred the racing mares which roared into town with their hooves clattering like castanets in a shapely gypsy dancer's hand. Meanwhile the carriage rumbled and delicately swayed with enormous speed. The mares' strides were huge and rapid, mesmerized by their own speed, they flaunted haughty attitudes, snorting and blowing through flaring nostrils. The coachman, always dignified and statue-still, controlled their strides impeccably. White foaming spittle would fly back from the mares' mouths; their ears playing with flickering rapidity. Their knees tilled the air high; their heads were raised on tall-arched necks. No wonder the sidewalks were lined with spectators, windows opened and filled with smiling faces when we rumbled through the asphalt streets of towns.

When foals were born, my father invited me to inspect them. They lay down on huge stacks of fresh hay with the mares circling them protectively. One morning, while inspecting a newborn colt, I was amused by his hopping around like a cricket overflowing with energy stimulated by our visit. I laughed at him and said to my father, "Give him to me, please."

And he answered, "He is yours."

Father instructed the estate steward to register the foal in my name. This is how I became a racehorse owner at age seven. He won the derby three years later and I got the large inscribed sterling cup. It sits in my display cabinet today. I sure knew how to pick them. But I was a greedy boy and I wanted a riding horse.

I went with my father to our racehorse breeding farm.

The young men herding the mares with their foals rode good-minded, well-meaning horses. I was hoping to have such a fine horse for myself one day. I was chatty and my father seemed deep in thought during our carriage ride home. But I still chatted to him amicably. My topic of conversation was about how nice it could be to get one of those herding horses to be mine, and have it moved up to the castle stable. Nearing home, Father seemed to have snapped out of his thinking and said, "What was that all about?"

"Of course it was all about you giving me a riding horse," I said.

So, being trapped next to me in a carriage, he seemed agreeable, "Go back to the horse farm and select one you like and then tell me about it," he said.

I did not waste much time and ordered the ponies and carriage for the next morning. I went out, selected a splendid looking herding horse. His name was *Csillag*, meaning star in English. His rider was proud that I had chosen him. The young herder felt honored and sad because he trained this horse; and now I was targeting the gelding for myself. At dinner I told my father: "I found a horse just right for me. It's a beauty with a kind disposition."

I listed all other imaginary attributes while my father ate and looked bored. At the end of my avalanche of thought, I finally took a breath or two. "He is yours, and I will have him sent up to the castle stables," Father said.

This is how I already owned two horses at the age of seven years. A "riding master" was assigned to teach and supervise me on my newly acquired horse. A rough, former cavalry sergeant, he ignored my superior rank and devoted himself to teaching me how to ride in the classical military style. He thought highly of discipline and endurance of pain. "Your lordship is not exhausted enough. How does your lordship imagine relaxing in the saddle without exhaustion?"

I submitted to all the rigors and pains of horseback riding and grew in prestige in his rough military mind. He even squandered compliments on me. "Your lordship would make a fine soldier."

19

As a child I had to join group lessons for children by well-known instructors at the nearby Artillery Barracks where there was a beautiful 19th century indoor riding school. The tone was militaristic and rough. We all understood that this was the culture of horseback riding. Riding is a martial art and its best representatives were military men. There, a loud and ill-tempered, military officer was drilling us. We were aged seven to about twelve years. We were all scared, mostly because of our respect for these military "divinities" in the center of the arena who knew everything. I got away with a lot because, as my peers pointed out, I was the "teacher's pet." I remember the officer in the center addressing one of my little nine-year-old riding colleagues, "Countess, you look like a hippopotamus with a liver disease."

The countess sniffled but was too scared to cry. She was very respectable for toughing it out.

My mother rode. She was an exceptionally beautiful lady and one who wore her beauty well; she seemed oblivious to it. Her horse was a wonderfully schooled dressage master, Tatar (Tartar in English.) She was "nailed to the bit" as my mother had very light hands and the horse "stayed in frame" regardless of the rider's skills. Tatar volunteered to be permanently "on the bit." My mother rode for pleasure, of course, and did not train horses nor compete. She looked her usual elegant self on this very tall, slender, chestnut-colored German horse. Mother rode under the shade of a black Girard hat augmented by a veil secured under her chin. She looked fabulous. One July morning, when the freshly harvested and threshed wheat was piled into straw bales scenting the fields, I rode with my governess in a fast carriage along the ancient oak forest just past the family crypt. My mother was cantering elegantly next to our carriage when her custodian, the wise Tatar, suddenly changed nature. He took off uncontrollably, darting off the road to the left into a harvested field of straw bales, several of which he jumped at a high speed. Then, Tatar somersaulted, throwing Mother a great distance. The horse lay motionless, dead. Mother got up, dusted herself off, adjusted her hat and smiled to reassure us that she was well. She felt loss of Tatar deeply. Autopsy showed that Tatar died of coronary aneurysm. She never owned another horse.

"LIBERATED" FROM EVERYTHING
WE OWNED

After those polite, tranquil and delicious days, the "Liberating and Glorious" Soviet Red Army arrived on November 30, 1944. They proceeded to liberate everyone from everything they owned. The process of "liberation" took many forms from the immediate detachment of one's wristwatch to the cumbersome and time-consuming dismantling of great wealth accumulated by four centuries of diligence and productivity. To steal and confiscate all my parents' and my possessions took the very diligent Communist dictatorship six years. It was completed when I was notified of the confiscation of our castle and everything else still registered in the family name in March of 1951. By then, I was fourteen and we were granted 48 hours to vacate our home. We took whatever could be fitted onto three trucks to Budapest where we had been allotted a portion of my grandmother's flat. We were also forbidden to enter the County in which our family had lived for centuries.

My parents were "liberated" from most of the thousands of livestock they bred and owned in 1945 by the "Glorious Liberating" Soviet Red Army. Among these were 86 racehorses of various ages and genders. Everyone was reduced to poverty as possession of private property became illegal. The poor were made destitute and so were the rich. The equality by poverty, scarcity of necessities, and fears consumed everyone's life. My mother quietly commented in Latin, *"Sic transit Gloria mundi."* (Thus passes the glory of the world.)

Then, she spent the rest of her long life not noticing the losses of her wealth, her status and her personal possessions. She never mentioned it. She was elegant.

I disregarded my governess' admonition, "Don't complain, and don't explain." Instead, I complained a great deal to my parents about the horrors of living in a totalitarian dictatorship. I bitterly predicted that the communist regimes would not be destroyed and would torment the world for millennia, ruling even longer than the Egyptian Pharaohs ever did. My father simply administered his tranquilizer, "Do not despair! Dictatorships always look indestructible until five minutes before they collapse. You will see much better days yet!"

Meritocracy was replaced by "politically correct," utterly politicized life, according to which individuals had only "collective value," measured by their value to the ruling communist regime. Merit was tolerated, even valued, when it was considered to benefit the government and its international prestige and appeal.

There came a day in 1952 when I was admitted to the riding academy in Budapest based on merit as experts saw it. By then, I had long been considered a skilled rider, with competition successes as a result of years of excellent instruction. The Riding Academy was hastily re-commissioned to replace the defunct famous Orkeny Riding Academy (See its history in chapter 7). I was admitted to the academic program as the youngest student ever in its history, due entirely to merit. In fact, my admission was potentially dangerous to those selecting me. I was already declared by the government "an enemy of the people" in our infamous "classless society." To select me for admission was dangerously in opposition to governmental policy. "Meritocracy" was replaced by politicized order in every aspect of life. It might help to understand that in Communist double talk "The People" really meant "The Communists." Therefore, enemies of the people were suspect, disarmed, helpless, and submissive enemies of the Communists. The "People's Republics" were really the Communists' Republics.

One thing was certain: We were all equal in poverty, degradation and deathly fear of governmental terror. As property was confiscated, the means of production and distribution of goods were nationalized, the only employer became the all-powerful state, and consequently, all citizens were enslaved. Many career advancements and advantages came to those participating in, and contributing to, oppression. Careers in cruelty were taking shape. The bitter joke made its rounds that "There are only three kinds of people in our society: those who were, those who are, and those who will be interred." Telling this "joke" could win one a sentence of ten years of hard labor if an informer were to hear it. When there was any trouble, the police were not called because they were not viewed as protectors but as persecutors at the command of oppressors.

Everything was politicized. Luckily for some of us, the artistic and athletic elite, selected mostly by talent, was subsidized to develop into propaganda units, providing the cultural and athletic successes as triumphant proof of communism's superiority. These tolerated "elites" became "ambassadors" for the "superiority of socialism." Fortunately for me, I was spotted as a fine equestrian prospect for socialism's' advertisement. At the same time, I was also an "enemy of the people" and as such, condemned to die eventually of hard and hazardous physical labor. We, the "enemies of the people," were barred from higher education and compelled to do only physical labor. The difficult task of constructing layers of lies commenced. As a sportsman I became a "state treasure."

Meanwhile, my father, the "class enemy in chief," had been interred in a concentration camp for three years. Some of my uncles and aunts were also languishing in hard labor slave camps. Camp and prison inmates were not accused, tried and condemned. These steps of bourgeois jurisprudence having been skipped, they went from capture directly to sentencing and never found out why. They were also routinely beaten and tortured. I took it upon myself to visit my father in exile for the two allowed days per year. Similarly, I was the only person allowed to visit one of my aunts in a concentration camp six times per year for 10 minutes each. The Academy permitted me these "sick leaves" from work without asking questions or expecting answers.

Without audible discussions, but rather, with nods and winks, a new biography was constructed for me, according to which I was "a simple son of the country" and "a young comrade in sport from close to nature in village life," "a hard working son of the villages." In the Age of Lies it mattered not that we previously owned three villages before we were liberated from them and banished into exile from our county.

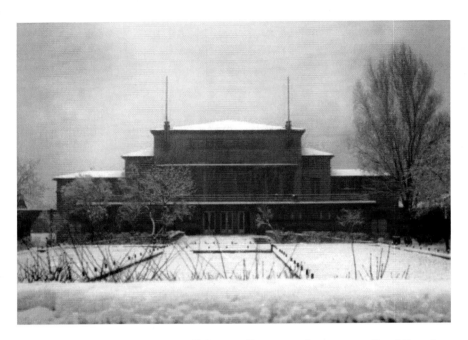

The Tattersal Riding Hall in Budapest photographed by the author in February,1954.

Horses saved my life as I emerged as a secret "darling of the regime" while half of my family was in the assembly line to death by hard labor. Ironically, I was admitted to the riding academy one year after my father was exiled to a concentration camp, preceded by repeated arrests and beatings without accusations. Once I asked him after his release from political prison how he was treated and he said, "A few years back these same fellows called me 'Jew-loving swine.' Now they called me 'blood-sucking Fascist swine.' Come to think of it, no one in prison addressed me as 'your lordship.'"

Even before my formal academic equestrian schooling began, I did my riding at the Tattersal in Budapest. It was named after Lord Tattersall, a great inspiration to nineteenth century racehorse breeding and competitions. I became aware of the Tattersal when my mother took me to visit my great Aunt Ilonka, in her villa on a wooded street on Rose Hill in Budapest. I was still very little and very impressed by her villa having a double garage, when most had none, so opulent that it could house her Rolls Royce and her elder son's Duisenberg. Uncle Peter explained to me that he needed the gigantic Duisenberg "to intimidate French drivers." He often drove to Paris. On the occasion of our visit, the footman informed my mother, "Her grace is riding at the Tattersal and will be back momentarily."

I was immensely interested by the fabulous word Tattersal. I instantly respected this unknown place because it lived up to the standards suitable to Aunt Ilonka's riding. Soon enough, the Rolls Royce drove to the portico and Aunt Ilonka hurried in with riding boots and silver-topped crop, smiling and kissing me loudly.

Some years later Aunt Ilonka told me this charming story. In June of 1941 Hungary entered the war by participating on the Russian front. The Americans declared war in December. Notice went out that anyone wishing to telephone the United States must place their call within 48 hours. Aunt Ilonka's younger son, Andrew, was living in New York, by then an American Citizen. Aunt Ilonka was being connected by transatlantic cable to New York when the Gestapo Agent "operator" yelled out to her a warning, "You may not talk in Hungarian, only in German, English, French or Italian. To which Aunt Ilonka replied, "You choose."

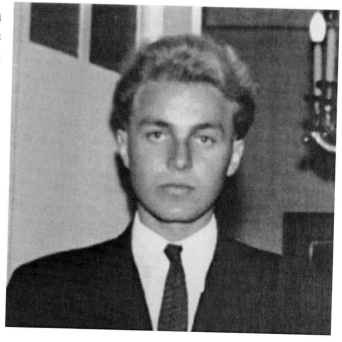

Charles de Kunffy during his second year at the riding academy

25

My Entrée into the Performing Arts

I had no time for sadness. On the backs of horses, all cares fell away from me. During most of my academic education in equitation I was still attending high school. It was during my teen years that even at the saddest times a mood of jollity would flood over me and propel me to a raucous hilarity. Overcome by such a mood I would wind up the gramophone and put on it a 78 vinyl record with the American Eddy Howard singing a jazz variation of "Ragtime Cowboy Joe." I bought this treasure on the black market, of course. At the time I did not speak a word of English but my parents had since they were children. This fabulous little ragtime song turned me into a song-and-dance performer without any warning. My parents comprised the unsuspecting captive audience as I began to sing along phonetically with Eddy Howard. I adored what I thought was the most beautiful American name, Eddy Howard. In my America-adoring mood, I imitated the sounds of this monosyllabic hectically rhythmic song. I pronounced my would-be English imitations well through the nose and secured the imitation of a "Western twang." Only the repeated phrase, "Ragtime Cowboy Joe" dropped out of my mouth in the original English version. The song was wizardly fast but I kept up with it in my ersatz English with impeccable fluency. As if this was not enough, I added some tap dancing and what I saw in American Films as "jazz dance" with gyrations to accompany my singing. I was slithering between the crowded furnishings of our living room, imitating Fred Astaire and other great dancers I had seen in American films during my childhood. My parents were in tears from laughter, saying, "You sing it better than the star on the recording. You should hire out to Hollywood."

This encouraged me to strut about with great swagger and to spin-around with pistol toting gestures as I imagined a cowboy would do it. My parents were grateful when I looked cheered up.

My parents especially enjoyed other scenes in my repertoire including my imitations of our cook during the "good old days." She was excellent but highly volatile. I had her dramatic encounters with the kitchen maids down pat. I rushed around

26

the living room as if it were our huge tiled kitchen filled with pots and pans. I was stirring sizzling sauces with imaginary spoons, meanwhile scolding the phantom kitchen maids, talking very fast in a high-pitched voice, punctuated by loud hick-ups. My parents were in stitches. We all loved the cook but my mother had to defend the kitchen maids valiantly, and had performed many diplomatic missions to the cook, until she could finalize cease-fires with the difficulty of an international peace conference. The cook was fierce when triggered by the maids. She was a redhead!

SCHOOLING AND PEERS

I was a private student, tutored at home during my elementary education. I took the final examinations at the municipal school. Our high school education lasted eight years from age ten to eighteen. After reaching my tenth year, I lived in Budapest during the school months and spent the holidays in the country at my castle. However, there were modifications to the routine tradition. Often we were given "coal holidays" by the government. This meant that there was not enough coal to provide heat. At the same time, the state-controlled media triumphantly proclaimed that coal production far surpassed that of the pre-war years. Consequently, schools were often closed for extended periods in the winter months. During these "coal holidays," I returned to the castle and its dreamlike beauty and comforts.

I had the great privilege to have been admitted to the only Catholic school tolerated by the Communist government. It was designated as a token propaganda piece to be confused by the Western press with "religious freedom." All the teachers were monks belonging to the most famous teaching order, the Piarists, founded in Rome by St. Joseph of Calazantium in the fourteenth century. I was admitted to this outstanding school because both my father and grandfather were alumni. Perhaps the pity the monks felt for us, "class enemies," barred from all academic high schools and ordered to enter trade schools instead, helped my admission. The priests were strict and excellent educators. Several had two doctoral degrees. I cheekily commented that they acquired two doctoral degrees for the sake of symmetry, in order to keep their balance and equilibrium.

My classmates thought me eccentric because I was admitted to the National Riding Academy, therefore I was excused from physical education classes and released early from school, and because I attended Wagnerian operas.

We must have been about 12 years old when my classmates discovered that I lacked two essential skills. I could not whistle, nor could I spit. They undertook to teach me both as they considered these skills essential to correct living. My classmates soon discovered that I was not an easy-to-train primate. The whistling was hopeless, even after frequent assistance by my peers placing their dirty fingers into my mouth to adequately deform my lips for the expected sounds. Nothing beyond some hissing passed my lips, and mercifully my friends gave up stretching my lips. They just pronounced me "impossible."

The spitting lessons also failed. My classmates suggested going to our balcony, four stories up, to allow the earth's center of gravity to help me spit all the way down to the street. Four of us gathered on our tiny balcony at the corner of our apartment and I was urged to spit out. Nothing was forthcoming. The wise suggestion to let saliva flow out of my mouth toward the street worked a little. From the fourth floor, my saliva dribbled down about half a floor and then vanished from sight. The result of these earnest hours of learning to whistle and spit was that I never acquired either skill and somehow grew old lacking them. When I was fourteen, we took a high school excursion to a painting exhibition of "Socialist Realism" designated by the Communists as the only "artistic" style allowed to be publicly viewed in our suddenly politicized lives. Anything seemed better than sitting in the classroom, filled with anxiety about failing to know our assignments. The monks were strict disciplinarians and academically demanding. Consequently, the predominant mood in the classroom was that of fear mixed with respect.

We walked from the school in pairs to the now non-existent exhibition hall on Erzsebet Square. Our Class Superior, a young priest, chaperoned us. We divided into polite little groups. My usual "fans" surrounded me. I took a look at the paintings hanging on the walls of the vast room and noticed their brainless depictions of "Socialist Realism" clichés of the "politically correct" muscular joys of building socialism and the banalities of waging "patriotic wars" to defend the "peace loving people" living in "fraternal societies." All the banalities of poster art depicting the prescribed propaganda were on display. Because my Great Uncle Lajos Kunffy was a famous painter and my mother, an accomplished sculptress, the trashy propaganda 'art' offended me.

I assumed a pretentious scholarly stance, with one foot forward, my chin resting on one fist and commenced to stare down these miserable products of politicized art. I improvised a pretentious monologue to mock the exhibition. I began to ventilate by rhythmically intoning the following monologue, preserved in the original Hungarian below as a friend carefully wrote it down at the time:

"A lagyan elmosodo szinek elenk fenyben hozzak ki a rajz plasztikajat. A tartalom es forma remek osszhangja, az a bagyadt szellemiesseg ami az egesz kepet oleli at, valoban modern es dekorativ."

"The softly blurred colors in vigorously vibrant light emphasize the linear plasticity of the picture. The superb harmony of the form and content, that limpid spirituality that embraces the entire picture, is truly modern and decorative."

Then I went on to the next "master piece" and repeated the same monologue. By about the tenth painting identically appraised, my group of followers was enormously swollen and they were all in various stages of choking from laughter. Only I remained unamused and scholarly. Thus, the viewing of "Socialist Realism" in art was a great success, and became a cherished memory. The young Priest, Class Superior, neglected to punish me for irreverence.

When I complained about our thankless fate to my theology professor, Dr. Medvigy (Father Michael), he wrote to me on the dedication page of one of his books, "Remember what Saint Theresa of Avila said: 'Let nothing bother you, let nothing dismay you. Everything passes. Patience gains all. God alone is enough.'"

This tranquilized my restless spirit. Some twenty years later we were friends and I addressed Father Michael as Brother Michael. We spent much time together in Rome, where he was summoned by Pope Paul VI. This great scholar's wish was to see the arrival of the new Millennium. He lived to see it and died, suitably, on Christmas Day 2000.

CHAPTER 2

MY DIVINE EQUESTRIAN TEACHERS

I had the greatest teachers, ever. Simultaneously three teachers observed and instructed me every day at the Academy. They even taught me prior to my admission which was based on their strong advocacy. I also had beneficial influences by other, "auxiliary" teachers that were woven into my equestrian life by circumstance.

All these brilliant instructors were "enemies of the people," "class enemies," "obstructionists," and "chained dogs of imperialism." As such, along with the other educated, capable and leadership elite of society, they were exiled from Budapest and forced into punishing physical labor.

As the communist government decided to advertise traditional Hungarian equestrian culture, they revitalized the National Riding Academy and lusted for a talented Olympic Team to be coached there. They seemed to have everything except knowledge and expertise. Classical horsemanship was not one of the qualifications for Communist Party membership. Rumor had it that at this time, the famous Czechoslovakian Olympic competitor of 1936, Frantisek Jandl, had the ears of the Communist potentates. He advised them to repatriate various "enemies of the people" to Budapest and to appoint them to establish and run the new National Riding Academy.

Therefore it transpired that all three of my teachers were relieved of their hard physical labor duties, "building socialism" in the countryside. All three had Doctoral Degrees. They were high-ranking military officers before the end of the war. After they graduated from the Hungarian Riding Academy of Orkeny, they were also schooled abroad in Tordiquinto and Pinerolo, Italy, in Hannover and Berlin, Germany, and at Wienerneustadt and at the Spanish Riding School in Vienna, Austria. They often competed internationally with great success.

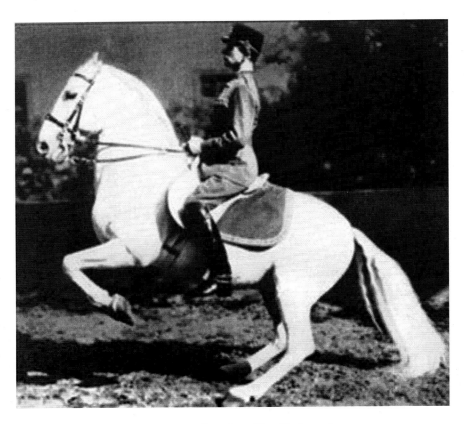

Geza Hazslinszky-Krull, levade

Colonel Dr. Imre Bodo was a world famous jumping rider. Among his many adventures was that he broke his neck in a jumping accident, recovered and continued competing and winning. After teaching me for about a month, he called me aside in the dressing room of the academy. He pulled me close. He intended to speak softly, "You don't remember me, do you?"

"No, Sir" came my quick reply as I scrutinized his sunburned, wrinkled face and sparkling, sad eyes.

"Well," he said. "Do you remember a black-out night in your castle at the end of the war? There was an air raid going on and a German anti-aircraft gun was mounted on a freight train at the railway station. They were firing at the British bombers that droned overhead. There was an officer playing Chopin Nocturnes at the piano in the ballroom by candlelight. Some of the ladies wept. That officer was me, and you were standing by the keyboard staring at my fingers working the keys."

Very humbled and moved by his recollection, I said, "Of course I remember you now, Sir."

"And how are your lovely parents?"

"My father is in a concentration camp and we are not allowed to see him."

Dr. Bodo nodded, as if to imply that he did not expect anything less meted out to a great man. I worshipped him and he looked after my riding education with near Divine benevolence.

Not everyone liked Colonel Dr. Jeno Kosa-Reznek because some thought him to be cold, distant, authoritarian, and harsh. I recognized in him all the military virtues that I had admired in my grandfather and in other officers in our large circle of friends. Dr. Kosa-Reznek was a superb instructor and coach. He knew his subject and communicated it well. His training methodology was impeccable. Our horses never refused fences. They did not stop, did not run out and did not break down. They were poor to mediocre quality horses that had survived the war. Our training results were the fruits of the knowledge and wisdom of our teachers.

Dr. Kosa-Reznek was a graduate of the Ludovica Academy, the Hungarian equivalent of America's West Point. He also graduated from the Hungarian Riding Academy at Orkeny and continued his education in Italy at Tor di Quinto and Pinerolo. He was never harsh with me because as the youngest in the academy, it was understood that I was to be the "teacher's pet." Jeno Kosa-Reznek was an internationally recognized authority on schooling horses, particularly in jumping. One of the greatest praise I ever received was when he declared, and did so quite often: "Charles has an exemplary jumping style. Most often perfect. He can also approach and depart jumps correctly."

I could siphon off some oxygen from comments like that. In the "good old days" Dr. Reznek won the coveted Coppa di Roma on his horse Merano. He was a very successful competitor in jumping and dressage. Academically impeccable, he could explain everything with great élan. Before he was ordered to instruct Hungary's best riders in 1951, he had been banished to "build socialism" as a pig herd at a huge hog-fattening farm at Nagyteteny, named for the despised communist dictator, Matyas Rakosi, a pink-skinned overweight tyrant, looking like a Yorkshire hog fattened for slaughter.

Dr. Reznek invited me to ride his Grand Prix horse one morning. He stood with hands on his hips, smiling, because I could not move his horse off the spot. After watching me suffer, he declared, "Your aids are 'too rude' for my horse to endure."

He emphasized "My horse is well-trained and cannot be expected to understand an unpolished youngster like you."

His horse finally lowered his dignity to my standards when I gave the softest aids: "Ride the air between your boots and his sides" was Dr. Kosa-Renznek's admonition.

At another time Dr. Reznek was polishing me up for a Prix St. George level test, which at that time had a "zigzag traversal" starting on the center line. This exacting half-pass work at the trot eluded me at the time, and having been officially a "teacher's pet," I received merely some sarcasm. Dr. Reznek said in a clarion voice, for all to hear, "Not all sideways disobedience is a half-pass."

Then, he drilled me for three quarters of an hour until my fit eventing horse drooped like a wash rag. I got the idea that I better perform this movement once really precisely if I want to survive. When I finally conquered the half-pass zigzag,

Dr. Reznek looked bored and said, "Dismissed."

I dismounted and handed my horse to my disapproving groom.

Dr. Pal Kemery was a graduate of the Spanish Riding School of Vienna. He was the oldest of the triumvirate of my mentors. At the 1936 Berlin Olympics, then Lt. Col. Pal Kemery rode Csintalan in the Dressage competition. His teammates were General Gustav von Pados on Ficsur and Colonel Laszlo von Magashazy on Tucsok. Dr. Kemery was small, until he sat on a horse with his long stretched legs and then he looked tall and lanky. He chain-smoked and acquired heart trouble and emphysema. He was a gentle and frail man and wore a pair of wire-framed glasses on his long aristocratic nose.

Dr. Kemery gave me the biggest equestrian compliment of my

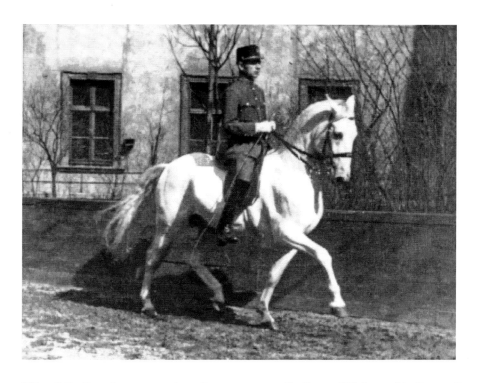

The fabulously correct and consequently beautiful equitation of Geza Hazslinszky-Krull inspired all of us to imitate him.

life. After I had trained my horse, Kormend for 4 years, Dr. Kemery asked me one day, "May I sit on your horse?"

I was astonished because he was then very frail even on solid ground and had not ridden for years. I was flooded by the honor of his request, jumped off Kormed and said, "But of course."

With my groom's assistance he settled on Kormend and already at the halt, he composed a splendid image. Then, off he went to walk, then collected trot, then collected canter and other pleasures. He made Kormend look inflated, unusually large, with dancing long legs, infused with magical energy. My horse was transported to a world of pleasant surprises and danced for joy. I thought my frail teacher made my horse resemble a spider. He looked as if he had a tiny, round, compact torso on long, slender legs.

From a canter Kormend dropped to a monumentally elegant halt like a snowflake alighting on the ground. Dr. Kemery dismounted and blinking from behind his wire-framed glasses, said, "If an old man with emphysema and heart disease can ride your horse with ease and pleasure, your training is laudable!" I almost melted on the spot.

Dr. Kemery, Dr. Bodo and Dr. Reznek were my friends and were admirers of my mother during the years when my father was imprisoned, deported and exiled. On one occasion when I was idling with Dr. Kemery on a bench, while he was smoking his eternal cigarette, he said, "You know the government put me, my wife and unmarried middle-aged daughter into a two room apartment with one tiny bathroom. My only remaining wish toward bourgeoisie decadence remains that I may live to see the day when I can again have my own bathroom."

Such a day never dawned on him.

The exemplary seat and kind nature of Colonel Geza Hazslinszky-Krull (1900-1981) was legendary. He was easily singled out to be the director and chief rider of the Royal Hungarian Spanish Riding School from 1932-1945, housed in a baroque palace adjacent to the Royal Palace of Budapest. Today the territory on which it stood is a vacant lot, a man-made desert in a re-awakening capital. Sometimes, I stand there looking into the nothingness of the sky that used to be blocked by the palace of the school. Geza Hazslinsky was the director of Budapest Spanish Riding School, the sister school of the shrine of classical equitation, the Viennese Spanish Riding School. His magnificent seat and imperceptible aids worked magic on any horse he rode.

Geza Hazslinszky-Krull was also classified in the communist "classless society" as a "class alien" and definitely an "enemy of the people." After he returned from many years of captivity in the Soviet Union, the Communists condemned him to perform hard physical labor and later to be a stable boy at the state stud at Mezohegyes. The new "aristocracy" of the "progressive" Communist Party members siphoned off his immense knowledge to run the stud farm without catastrophes, regardless of their ignorance of horses.

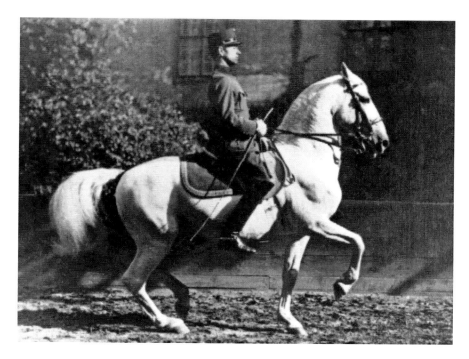

Geza Hazslinszky-Krull, piaffe.

It took Stalin dying and Khrushchev posturing as benefactor, to allow the equestrian genius, Hazslinszky, to teach again.

Colonel of the "old" army, Hazslinszky spotted me at an equestrian training camp at the Koros River and volunteered to teach me intermittently, whenever possible from 1954-1956. For the Communists he was a "caricature of a gentleman." That meant, of course, that he was an impeccable gentleman. He retained his slender figure and an officer's deportment, and managed to dress in tattered old clothes looking elegant and suave.

Amusing stories were told about him by two of his eminent students of the pre-war years in the Royal Hungarian Spanish Riding School, Andras Bondor and Imre Magyar. These magnificent riders volunteered to be my mentors in the Academy, where a hierarchy of teaching existed. In addition to our instructors, well-skilled mentors were training "school horses" to higher levels and then allowed us to ride these superbly trained horses under their tutelage.

Bondor and Magyar were fabulous riders and their horses became my professors. Both men drank a lot. This showed only on Magyar, however, he could ride better drunk than most of humanity can do soberly.

Among the Hazslinszky anecdotes, stories of kindness and charity figured highly. As a high ranking officer and the director of the Hungarian Spanish Riding School, Col. Hazslinszky had many sub-ordinates. These soldiers approached him toward the weekends with requests to ask him for a "leave" on account of a dying relative, usually an aunt or a grandmother. No visitations to male relatives, of course, during a war, because males died a "natural death" on the battlefields.

The clever Hazslinszky could sense by the approach of a recruit the purpose of his visit and without looking up from his desk would address the soldier: "You may visit anyone dying for three days and then report back to me."

The broadly smiling youngsters jauntily walked away from his presence. He was all heart and kindness to everyone. Even the Communists in authority over him admired his character and appreciated his sweet nature. He was extricated from Hungary by Prince Bernhard of The Netherlands who requested him for the Royal Stables from none other than Nikita Khrushchev. He was the only authority that could not be denied a request to permit a Hungarian citizen to emigrate by the Hungarian Government. This, in itself, speaks volumes of the "independence" of Soviet Satellite States, such as Hungary, where only the Soviet dictator had the authority to release an important Hungarian expert to emigration.

The "punch line" is that Geza Hazslinszky was not just the Leonardo da Vinci, the Michelangelo and the Rafael of riding, but an inspiration of how to remain a gentleman even in hell.

I received very few, incidental lessons from Gabor Bukkhelyi, a dear friend of my parents. As a young officer, he became a friend when he was stationed at the artillery barracks at Tolna, our home town. Many of the young officers came regularly to our dinners, hunts and grand balls with their wives. Gabor was a bachelor with a deep, gravelly voice, and a kind, contemplating glance that hid his uproarious sense of humor. One day, this daring rider rode out to our castle and was offered the usual selection of drinks and refreshments: he departed late, rather drunk. That gave Gabor the excuse to ride back out to our castle on the following day to apologize for his unseemly behavior. This resulted in him becoming drunk again and he continued to ride out daily to apologize for his behavior the evening before, which he continued to pursue without regret. My parents broke the cycle of these visitations by retaining him as an overnight guest, to "sleep it off." Thereafter there was no reason to canter to our house and get drunk again. Gabor was always forgiven because of his great goodness and charm.

He visited us again in Budapest when I was at the Academy and told an amusing anecdote. He was taken to a slave labor camp by the Communists, to "build socialism" by mining stone until "death by labor" would end the existence of this "enemy of the people." During heavy labor, he overheard fellow prisoners telling the anecdotes about their past. One was boasting of having had a commanding officer that could drink a bottle of liquor and still canter miles on his horse. The hero of this story of drunkenness was Gabor, overhearing the anecdotes while mining the stones with a smile. He was legendary for his heroism as a soldier, and the many peasant boys, now also designated "class enemies" in slave labor camps would talk about him, not recognizing in this gaunt, starving inmate the swaggering hero of their past. Gabor would seldom visit us but I always had a shot of plum brandy for him. He was a superb rider and a kind teacher.

Sandor Balint was hired to teach lessons to young riders in the late evening hours after school or work. He had been one of the greatest distance riders before the communists forced this "class enemy" to repair typewriters in a large factory. He was assigned to take us on Sundays to great cross-country rides, his specialty. We trotted out of the city onto country dirt roads in pairs; he always asked me to ride to his left. My horse matched the rhythm and tempo of his, and we trotted side by side on our horses that moved like a well-trained pair of carriage horses in front of a Landau. Sandor also knew my family socially. He could talk about many things other than horses. He was a philosophical man and very modest.

CHAPTER 3

MY GROOMS

I had three grooms that attended to my horses. There was an "old one" that was then younger than I am now. He was excellent. We called him Uncle Jozsi. He commuted from a distant suburb at impossibly early and dark hours by a horribly overcrowded commuter train. As so many people did then, he existed rather than lived. He loved only two things: caring for horses and assisting me. When we were very far from the rest of humanity, and could almost imagine that no one was overhearing us, he would say, "I know that you are a gentleman and I will never betray you. When I get up in the middle of the night to come to work, I do it gladly because I know that I am going to please a gentleman." He was very small, but very strong. He looked worn by long and hard physical labor. He was stingy with words, like most peasants. When he said something, it was worth hearing. His wife appeared a few times, usually to bring some food. She was much younger than Uncle Jozsi and very good-looking. Everyone just wondered how on earth he had a wife so attractive. After work, he did not shower and change as the other grooms did. When I asked him why he did not shower, he just said, "If I do not stink of horses and manure I lose my seat on the commuter train and have to hang on the train's steps all the way home. When I stink, people give me room." I thought it was a well thought out plan.

Another of my grooms was Imi, a teenager. He always smiled, had an incredible sense of humor and often slipped into the role of a stand-up comic. I was a very grateful audience and I loved to laugh at his stories. He was funny, even in the smallest ways. When he saddled my large-girthed Sator, he made a running commentary about my fat mare that was so funny that I had to laugh until I sat down from weakness. He had one story that was neither funny, nor amusing. He was a war orphan. He had been collected from the rubble of a ravaged Budapest after its infamously brutal six-week-long siege. He was starving, home-less and a scavenger when he was found and taken over by the authorities. He, with thousands of others, was given shelter in an orphanage. When the Communists finally took over all institu-tions, they devised for these orphans a merciless indoctrination program, none of which took root in my groom. I questioned him about his memories. He did not remember ever having parents. He said that he remembered with some affection, something like loving, a young-looking man that played the violin all the time instead of playing with him. We both presumed that the violin-ist might have been his father. He had absolutely no memory of any woman. He often jested to me, off-handedly, in a way that seemed sometimes irrelevant. One of these proclaimed, "I would die for you if you ever needed rescuing." I believed it. Luckily, proof was never needed.

My third groom was Pisti, also very young and very shy. He did excellent work. He could clean horses and tack better than anyone else. His colleague, the orphan Imi, used to sneer, "His is not cleanliness anymore; he is maniacal." Pisti seemed touched when the horses he groomed were winning. He had my permission to ride my horses sometimes when we were not available due to sickness or absences to shows. He rode well and had very good hands, the calling card of a good rider!

Two years before my schooling was completed two more grooms were accepted at our stables. They were not assigned to my horses. Both were aristocrats, recently released from So-viet slave-labor camps. Of course, they were marked for life by their sufferings, not just physically but also emotionally. The well-known symptoms included utter silence. In slave camps you learn, obviously, that thoughts may still be uncensored and are safe, but that utterances cause suffering and death. These muted gentlemen worked harder than anyone else in the stable staff. They lifted the heaviest loads, labored at the hardest tasks and made all of that look easy. They seemed to have enjoyed bru-tally heavy labor as if on vacation. They said nothing. They never looked happy or sad. They seemed to have been staring inward and listening to silence. My relatives that survived concentration camps behaved identically. These gentlemen were also extraordinarily clean and orderly. They reminded me of my mother's admonition, "We must survive these interesting times not only with life but with our culture."

In various stables on the grounds of Tattersall worked other aristocrats that were condemned to physical labor by decree. Not many people could choose their employment in Communist countries. After all, there was only one employer, the State, and it had plans for everyone, mostly at odds with individual hopes and aspirations. One stable boy that I will call Lajos was an intellectually brilliant and highly cultured young aristocrat "punished," as usual, for having dared to be born to titled parents. But his additional "crime" was that his younger sister, who was incidentally previously engaged to one of my uncles, now lived in New York and was married to an "American bloodsucking capitalist."

Yet another aristocrat working as a stable hand had the calloused hands of a laborer, a kind, sunburned face, a sturdy body strengthened by hard labor and a very severe haircut suitable for a soldier, delivered by a cheap barber. Incidentally, she was a lady. Everyone adored her. She was a well-known equestrian star and socialite in the Good Old Days, for she was none other than Erzsebet Keresztes, known to the "inner circle," which also included me, by the nickname "Muci." She was Hungary's finest lady jump rider, while in dressage the Arch Duchess Augusta excelled before the Soviet occupation. Muci carried the heavy cross of a "politically incorrect" pedigree. Her father was the famous General Keresztes, a military hero and adjutant to the Emperor Francis Josef. Her mother was the Austrian Princess Schwarzenberg, member of one of the three families that were wealthier than the Emperor himself.

Now, however, Muci was an exemplary stable hand and was permitted to train a few horses but not to compete on them. She had the inner elegance that kept her contented with her fate because she was allowed to be with her beloved horses. She appeared physically strong but even stronger was her uncomplaining spirit. Every day she would change from grubby working clothes to her riding attire and began her training duties.

42

Some of us watched her riding for hours. She was the only woman laborer at the stables and blended into her harsh circumstances by behaving as any of the strong male laborers. Grateful for any kindness, she still refused her colleagues' constant deference to her gender and high birth. I reveled in the sights when my practiced eye observed her way of putting on her Viennese doeskin gloves before a ride, and I watched her striding in her custom made, cognac-brown riding boots that glistened like mirrors, as they all shouted, "Princess!"

I never suffered from being in bad company. My world was filled with miraculously fabulous people, both titled and commoners. We were all equal in our suffering from poverty and merciless oppression.

For a while, our stable master was an informer who watched us, and as expected, reported weekly to the authorities. He wasn't very bright and one time, I overheard a member of the secret police utter in half-tones, "The man is not the brightest light bulb." Everyone "could smell him a mile away" and gave him wide berth. An old professional stable manager, now demoted, did the actual running of the stables and he ensured the welfare of the horses.

CHAPTER 4

JUMPING BY DESIGN

A skinny little blond boy in a well-tailored jacket that was somewhat large for him entered the covered arena of the Tattersall. His boots were much too large for him but they were exceptionally beautiful, having been custom-made in Vienna for his mother. His riding crop had a conspicuously large gold tip, engraved with his monogram under the Baronial crown. It had been a Christmas gift from several years prior by his Great Aunt Ilonka, who was since then, killed in the war. That boy was me.

I was entered into my first open jumping competition. I was expected to learn from the experience and was not expected to out-compete the seasoned adult riders in the class. I sat on a sixteen-year old chestnut gelding, named Vetek ("Sin" in English) and with my eleven years was much the horse's junior. The older partner was selected to give courage and confidence to the younger one. My horse survived the war in Budapest. Others were killed and often eaten by a starving population during the six-week long cruel siege on the Capital.

My much-admired Vetek was a jumping schoolmaster. He had been jumped far too much by the military where he was used to teach young recruits that were drafted. Consequently, he was "hanging at the knees" and had his font legs so deformed that they looked like the legs of a baroque piano. When I stood him up properly four square, facing the judge, his front legs quivered continuously. I saluted smartly with my whip, as required by protocol, and received a round of applause from the spectators. Prior to riding a course over fences, we were required to walk it and devise a suitable strategy. At the very least, I was expected to describe each jump, in the correct order, adding the description of each turn or other necessary action. It was something like the following example: "Start on right lead canter, take the first, inviting birch fence, land on left lead and jump the triple bar, right lead landing, hairpin turn and rally strongly to the red stonewall, remain highly alert because along the next wall is the double, between them, sit down and push, must land on right lead, on the diagonal is the vertical single bar with 'too much air underneath it' and the horse should approach from excited collection, etc." My coach listened with amusement and occasionally corrected or added to my strategies.

The whistle sounded and off I went with Vetek to our confidence building round. After the sixth jump, my memory failed me and there were six more fences to find in the right order. This amounted to a valid scientific proof that one does not have to be old, senile or have Alzheimer's to draw an absolute blank. I lost my memory of the course and Vetek puzzled about my taking him down to a trot. He had fine enthusiasm for jumping and seemed disappointed with the brevity of this course. Some buzzing, sighing and giggling sounds came from the spectators' bleachers. My memory refused to recover. I think I may have even forgotten my own name if asked then. I trotted to the judge's seat, halted my horse smartly, saluted with my gold tipped whip to signal my withdrawal from contest and exited in a hurried canter.

When I was schooled in the art of classical horsemanship, all of my teachers agreed on the basic principles about the nature of the horse, the goals of training and the legitimate methods by which these goals could be pursued and achieved. Those who understood the subject, found nothing controversial about any of the principles that were based on rational observations by hundreds of thousands of pragmatic equestrians of the past.

All principles issued from the fundamental precept: the love of the horse was paramount. Commitment to correct training and equestrian ethics was animated by this emotional commitment. Cynics can indulge themselves by saying that the so-called love for horses was based on pragmatic self-interest. Horses were of great value and owning well-schooled ones extended their serviceable life and, in turn, glorified the trainer/rider. Indeed, longevity, good health and splendid enhancement of the horse's athletic potential were the guiding principles to schooling. Kings and emperors wanted to be memorialized enthroned on horses in bronze or stone for public viewing.

Horses elevated the rider above the pedestrian crowds and raised the rider to ethical heights appropriate for leaders epitomizing strengthened character and profuse virtues.

Young horses were trained to become all-around equine athletes. Knowledgeable, systematic and gradual physical and mental improvement developed the proper strength and skills to carry the weight burden of the rider without discomfort, pain or breakdown. The first three years of training, the so-called campagne school, was designed to build a superb athlete. Emphasis was put on cross-country riding over highly varied terrain and on diversification of tasks. Cavaletti work and jumping, especially multiple combinations of fences were pursued regularly to enhance the horse's athletic strength from which, the athletically enhanced natural gaits emerged. It was with the essential help of cross-country work, cavaletti and combination jumps that horses came to the rider's aids, and became supple, elastic, energetic, rhythmic and powerfully impulsive.

Everything was considered "dressage work." Sliding down an embankment, jumping a triple bar, leaping up a bank or galloping fast on a forest lane were all considered necessary extensions of dressage exercises. All work, especially jumping, needed quick, precise and decisive rider control and therefore all training had to be done "on the aids." All exercises had to be done with the horse longitudinally flexed; the horse surrendering control of his haunches to the rider and remaining responsive to the leg, seat and rein aids. Specialization of horses was for competition purposes and was based on the horse's aptitude, inclination and even pleasure. After three years of gradual, basic training of the equine athlete, his genetic talents become obvious. Our goal was to nurture and develop the horse's genetic potential.

Work at the canter was emphasized. We were assigned to "canter-in" (Eingaloppieren in German) our young horses. Canter being the most natural and archaic of the gaits, the horse gains his impulsion, his elasticity, his strength and his pleasure in this gait. My teachers believed that "Canter builds the horse, so that the trot can use him up." We simply did not condition horses at the trot. Canter was king and horses needed it for improved respiration and cardio-vascular health. On all my jumping photos, one can see the results of outstanding training with a wide variety of breeds of backyard horses moved over fences in exemplary style. We were taught that the horse can, and should be, ridden with great precision to the take-off for the obstacle, and depart from it with rider's instruction. Over the fence, in flight, the horse merely needed impeccably balanced companionship and freedom from the rider.

Highly varied jumping exercises honed both rider and horse the necessary skills for harmonious precision. In praise of the outstanding education I received from all of my instructors, I was never bucked off or thrown by a horse. Obviously, I did not provoke them and when they needed to jump and take flight, I had a balanced and adhesive seat to stay on.

"The safest place is always on the horse, never on the ground!" was a frequent admonition. During the thousands of jumps I did with eight horses and counting each pole or fence, we never ran-out or stopped. We did only what horses were prepared to do with success. I went down with my horses four times. They were all jumping accidents caused by slipping at the take off from soft, muddy, slippery puddles.

I rode my horses on a simple bridle with a jointed snaffle and without any mechanical gimmicks. No standing or running martingales. No double bridles, no tie downs, simply nothing more than a rider. Yet, I had absolute control over our performance. How did I control a strong event horse that was fed 34 pounds of oats a day with Herculean strength? Did he pull out my arms? No, my horses were on the aids in lightness.

I always strived to be in harmonious balance with the horse. Torso low, rounded lumbar back and chest deep over the horse's forehand in aerodynamic unity. The seat, the pelvic structure remained close to the saddle to support a fluent change of the center of gravity, especially for smooth landing. Accompanying the horse, as if one were part of his structure, was demanded for undisturbed balance. Knees deep and closed, feet parallel with the horse's sides and well-flexed ankles with heels down remaining motionless during flight. A straight line leading from the rider's elbows through the reins to the horse's mouth guaranteed his freedom to navigate with his neck.

"It is not the rider that jumps up to clear the fence. It is the horse. The rider seeks quiet unison with a horse that is permitted to be the athlete."

One heard constant advice with important principles repeated. The coach shouted into the megaphone, "Stop moving around. You disturb the horse. You jeopardize his balance!" or yelling out, "You tell him on which lead to land. That is not the horse's option!" There was an inexhaustible fountain of ideas about how to control horses before and after the jump. On the most primitive level, one trotted to a cavaletti, struck one stride of canter and then leapt. The trot had to have correct impulsion, collection, posture, throughness and suppleness. The one stride of canter had to be with vigor, energy and straightness. Everything was academically designed and practiced until executed with near perfection. The tasks were clearly set and riders applied themselves to execute properly. Praise was earned.

Whatever the training tasks, we had to execute them within a very precise rhythmic profile. All riding was musical and we counted mentally, in silence as if riding a train, clicking on old rails. My strict teachers admonished me "You don't have to be smart to ride well. Even the most stupid person can count 'one, two, one, two' and keep rhythm. Are you able to cope with that difficult task?" came the sarcastic scolding. At the end of one of these lessons, I approached my admired Dr. Kosa-Reznek and dared to say, "Uncle Jeno, counting 'one-two' is not enough. I need to count 'one, two, three, four, five, six, seven' very evenly to really establish rhythm. For just drilling the 'one, two' can be done very fast and ruin the balance of the horse."

He thought for a minute and said, "I agree. Never thought if it. From now on, count to seven."

One may observe, however, with sadness, the shabby equipment (tack) on the horses and the shabby clothing of the rider. In the "dictatorship of the proletariat" consumer goods and stores to sell them disappeared. Our boots and britches were "issued" by the military upon requisition. We did not have private funds for buying riding attire, and money could not even find such "exotic" luxuries as boots and britches in the "nationalized" stores. There was an official propaganda culture of hatred against any hint of elegance. Boot and saddle makers vanished into the labor camps. Sport Clubs issued shirts to their members that never needed ironing. Casual shabbiness was accepted as riders' "uniform."

It is important to note that we were not required to ride with helmets. In fact, I do not recall seeing any helmets anywhere in Hungary in those years. Even before the war, riders wore no helmets. Military and police officers rode in uniform and wore their hats but they were never helmets. That does not mean that bareheaded riding is a good idea. In fact, riders should always ride with helmets! Safety first!

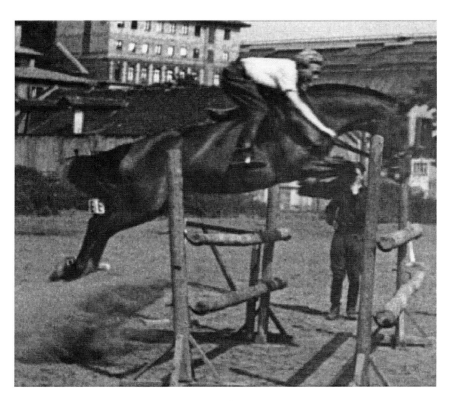

Sator, in training at the Tattersal.

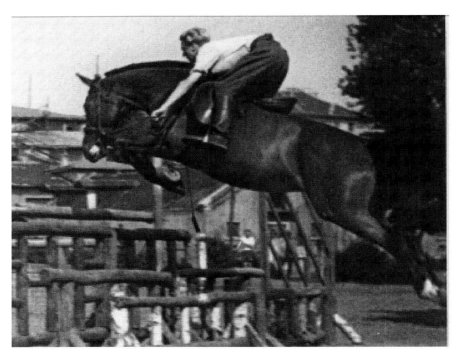

Sator, my only mare, had the power and bravery for jumping.

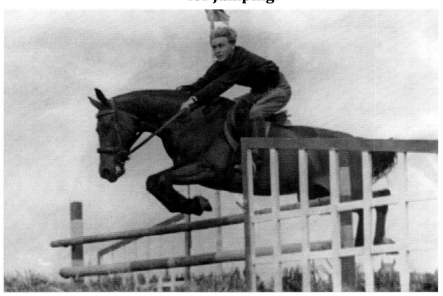

Sator's conformation made jumping difficult for her.

CHAPTER 5

MY HORSES, THE GENIUSES

SATOR

There was an unlikely pair of mares pulling freight in a peasant cart, bringing sacks of oats, bales of hay and straw to the riding academy. We saw them every day and those little mares were duly ignored. The one, pulling on the right, was unusual looking, having very large and strong hindquarters. But she also had short and steep shoulders and an ugly short neck, attached very low. She had features that would have been amusing in a comic book drawing. Curiously, she paid a lot of attention every time she spotted me on the cobblestones of the stable yard. I had sugar cubes in my sticky pockets and always gave her one when she stood in front of the wooden cart with her sadly hanging big

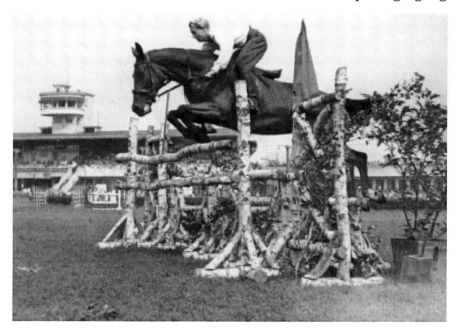

Sator extending her topline better.

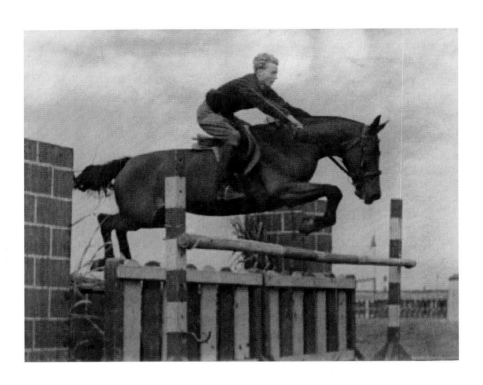

These pictures illustrate her gradual improvement
of elasticity and style.

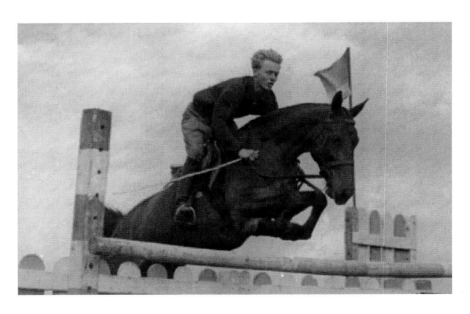

head.

Coincidental to these times was a committee selecting horses for us to train. I jeopardized my "prestige" in recognizing suitable horses at the age of fourteen by asking for this strangely constructed mare. Heaven knows there were shortages of everything in a communist country, even of available horses. I got her unhitched from the cart and she was assigned to me for riding. When I sat on her first, I thought she did not even feel like a horse. One saw too much ground, as her neck and shoulders did not fill the usual visual space. Her overbuilt croup made me feel like I was sitting on a slide. She looked permanently fat on any diet. She was chunky, ugly, badly configured and I called her "My Little Meat." However, her real name was "Sator," which means, "Tent" in English. A riding colleague of mine joked that if she were to have horns, she might be mistaken for a pig, meaning that she looked like any other species but a horse.

She became a sensational jumper, documenting the glo-

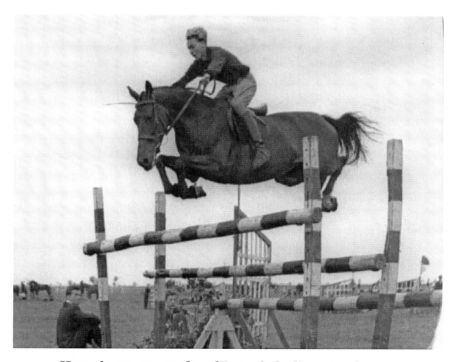

Here is an example of Sator's helicopter jump.

ries of our knowledgeable, systematic schooling system. She bounced over fences like a rubber ball. Because of her short and low neck she could not navigate too well. Often, when the jumps were high and wide, she took it like a helicopter: Straight up from a trampoline position, followed by a seemingly eternal hesitation above the jump with her legs tightly jerked up, providing me with a feeling of unwelcome hovering, and then plummeting straight down on the other side of the fence with her neck almost disappearing between her knees. She did not stretch her neck and her head remained inexplicably vertical above the fences. Many of her jumps were a scary experience.

But let me brag that the coaching and our training was so correct that none of the horses – often of terribly poor quality – "ran out" or stopped in front of a fence. My coaches, all three of them, deserve credit for such flawless record in expert schooling of horses and riders. Sator trusted my choice of jumps and was used to dealing with the fences because they were suitable to the level of her strength and her skills. She simply did not take poles. After clean courses we had to ride off on a second round of jumps for time advantages to determine placing. My chunky, small-striding mare was so nimble that she could land off the fence, spin, take a stride and execute the next fence faultlessly and we often won with the best time. She could turn on a dime and take a big fence without needing space for a lengthy approach. She could repeat her stunt to land off a fence, spin, stride and jump big and clean up the class. I could hear spectators laugh and giggle at her performances. The little fat mare was a nimble and comic crowd pleaser. She was also courageous and devoted. She often saved my neck.

The joke was that Sator was the only living thing aware of the competition calendar. We often got very short notice to get ready and compete somewhere. While we were kept ignorant of competitions in the year ahead, Sator somehow knew the competition dates. She was always in season for every competition. Despite her condition, she still jumped impeccably. But she pinned her ears back to every horse in the warm up arena and conspicuously squealed. I was very embarrassed and passed other riders, saying, "Pardon me."

Finally, Sator floats with neck stretched and head extended.

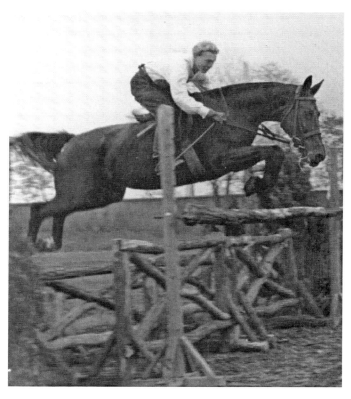

Sator was a spectators' favorite. In an equestrian country everyone could discern that she was not born for stadium jumping. I was also a crowd pleaser on account of my youth and unusually blond hair. The two of us usually got great applause just for entering the arena. This obliged us to pay back the applause by winning.

Years later, at a large championship show on Margaret Island, I won three big jumping events that had many entries. Two of those wins were with Sator and we were heartily congratulated by my coach. That was when I bragged, "It is not difficult to win after dancing all night."

Well, my coach heard that report with great interest and said "For irresponsible and unsportsmanlike behavior and for a special enthusiasm for nightlife, I assign you to overnight stable duty for a week." He walked away from me. I had seven nights at the stables to contemplate my duties toward horses, sport and the arts.

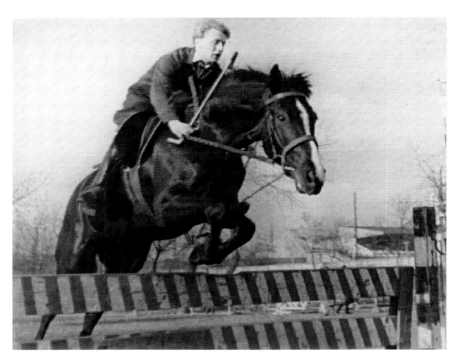

Hortobagy in training.

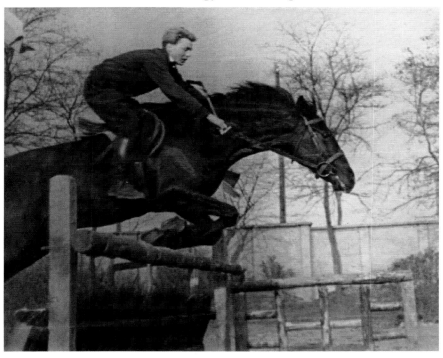

HORTOBAGY

This black gelding was tall, elegant and eminently photogenic. I met him on a terrifyingly cold winter evening. A pitch-black night had descended early and we exercised horses on straw thinly-spread over the icy ground. A bitter wind penetrated our clothing and the cold visited the interior of our riding boots. Credit went to us riders for balancing the horses impeccably on the ice-skating rink. I remember an interminable, steady, rhythmic trot work, occasionally changing directions. Our invisible instructor's voice came from the pitch dark at the center of our circle. He spoke wisely and interestingly about the theory of riding. His topics were more suitable to a classroom than to an iced-over arena. His lectures were brilliant. Being on horseback while he talked, we felt the meaning of his words transferred to practical experience. On this particular night, the instructor was Sandor Balint, a well-respected distance rider in the good old

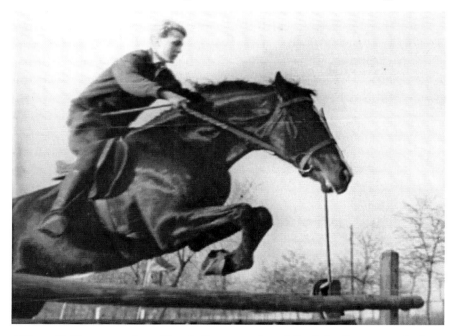

The gliding master, Hortobagy using his fabulous neck for navigation. He jumped smoothly and silently like a thief.

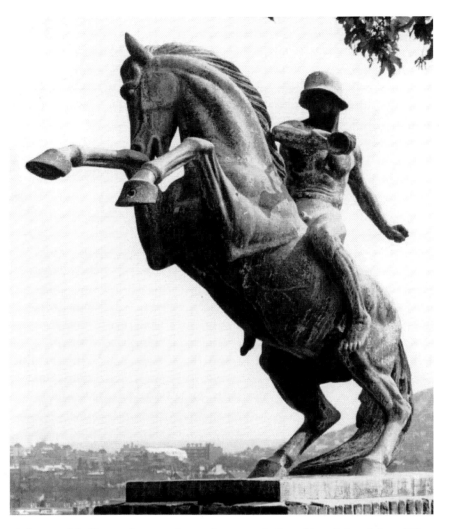

A beautifully animated warhorse defending his rider. They seem to live for one another in the midst of peril.

days, and a war hero. Now he was a typewriter repairman and, for an extra pittance he worked evenings teaching at the riding school. He confessed to me that he would have taught us even if he were not paid because he sorely missed being with horses and riders.

In early spring, the elegant Hortobagy, suspended from my adhesive and steady seat, floated at a gravity-defying extended trot; we attracted the attention of a famous and brilliant

58

sculptor. He was scouting the "horse world" for suitable models for equestrian sculptures. He had received a commission from the State for a public monument to commemorate military heroism. Hortobagy and I were selected to be his models, on account of the beauty of my elegant black horse. We were photographed a great deal. Fortunately he searched the illustrations in the National Archives for an image of a horse rearing. I had to pose shirtless to show off my then splendid abdomen, shapely pectorals, wide shoulders and slender waistline.

The resulting monument, generously idealizing my physique, hopefully did not become the envy of Michelangelo's David, idling in Florence. Hortobagy and I had inspired the large monument, placed on the shady Arpad Setany promenade in Budapest. By the time it was completed, I lived in California.

While I was "monumentalized" as my friends sarcastically teased me, I was required to go to the sculptor's atelier for sittings. In addition to sculpting us for the commissioned monument, the artist made a smaller composition with me on horseback – this time fully clothed – and the second statue, "A boy with his horse" now stands in a small public park along the

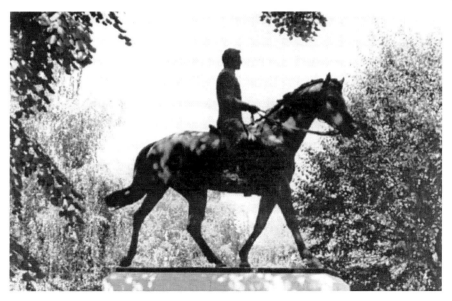

The author as "a boy with his horse"

59

Danube.

These two equestrian bronze statues are still on display to a strolling public oblivious to my identity. The public hardly ever glances at these monuments.

The bureaucratic elite discovered me on horseback and the adventures continued. This time the riding academy was ordered to release me for riding scenes in films. I was "requisitioned" by the Ministry of Culture from the Ministry of Sport in the eternally hierarchic structure of a dictatorship in which only the state's interest mattered and the individual was not consulted about his wishes.

We were not hired; instead, we were requisitioned, allotted and transferred. The needs and the will of the individual were, of course, ignored. Not that I would have objected to being

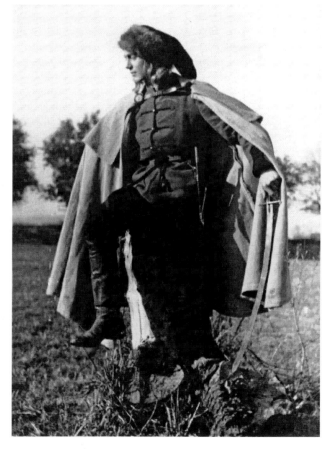

In late 17th-Century patriotic Kuruc fighter's uniform for the film 'Rakoczi's Lieutenant.'

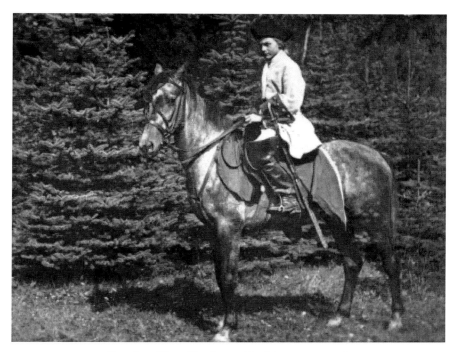

**In the film 'Rakoczi's Lieutenant'
here in the enemy Labanc uniform.**

in movies, even if my role were to be the third squatting midget in the fourth ditch on the left. So it transpired that I was shipped over to the mountain resort of Lillafured for several weeks – on loan, as objects ought to be – to be an extra in the film: "Rakoczi's Lieutenant."

When the film opened, my riding peers rushed me to the advertising poster, yelling, "Look, you are announced!" and they pointed to the poster that proclaimed in large letters the names of the film stars, and with tiny, hardly discernible script at the bottom of the poster admitted, "And also hundreds of others." My peers leered, "And there you are!"

I was also asked to be an extra in three additional movies, filmed in Budapest. In one of them, I stood with my horse most of the time at the garden gate of a socialism-loving girl that preferred driving tractors to having decadent fun with young men.

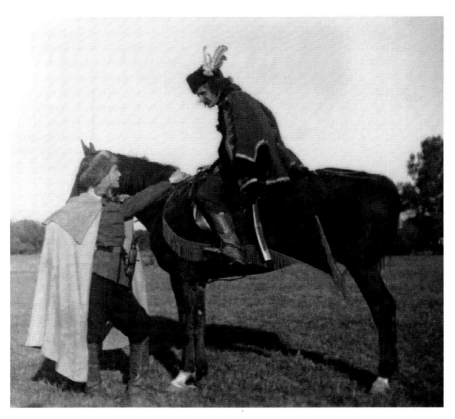

**de Kunffy in Kuruc fighter's uniform (left)
in the film 'Rakoczi's Lieutenant.'**

Another film, the title translating to 'Electing a King for a Day,' chronicled the life of Sandor Rozsa, a Hungarian version of Robin Hood. I wore a nineteenth century peasant outfit and was jumping over fences; one was a dining table.

Film career aside, Hortobagy was not merely a "film star" and a famous "model" but also a smooth jumper. His takeoffs to fences were like the floating ascensions of supersonic jets. He landed with the same finesse. He was like a smoothly landing glider. Between jumps he also felt as if he were skating on ice, moving seamlessly. His canter was the smoothest I have ever felt, and his flying changes were barely discernible.

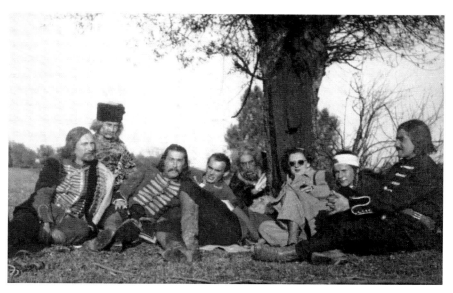

Actors at rest during filming: The fourth from the left is the famous Istvan (Pista) Hegedus (see page 107).

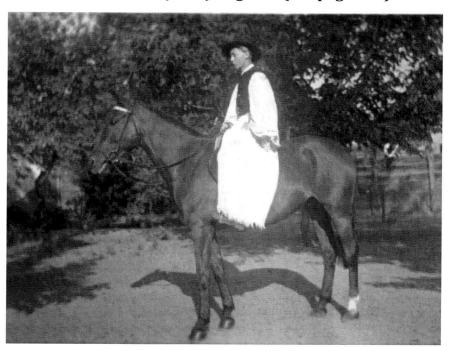

In costume for 'Electing a King for a Day.'

GADARA

Andras "Bandi" Bondor tutored me often on his well-schooled horse, Gadara. He was a gelding with great talent for jumping but was shown mainly in dressage, where he shined. Bondor, having been a rider of the Hungarian Spanish Riding School, had dressage expertise. Gadara performed all of the Grand Prix movements, including piaffe and passage as did another of Bondor's wonderfully schooled horses, Helyes. Helyes, meaning *charming* in English, was generously offered to me for lunging and experiencing piaffe, passage, flying changes in sequences and pirouettes. I had to do flying changes "a tempo" with Helyes on the lunging circle and the "professor" did it while I was in a daze. Helyes was so supple that I was complaining to Bondor "You de-boned him." He felt too soft to have a skeleton. Sitting on him felt as if one were sitting in a tub of chocolate pudding. Helyes was the color of chocolate without any markings.

Returning to the story of Gadara, there came a day when Bondor thought well of my jumping to request of the coaches to assign Gadara's jump work to me. For me, Gadara was the Rolls Royce of jumpers. Had I been brainless, he would have still executed a clear course. He was one of only three horses that I jumped on courses at the international height of 160 cm. Feeling strong, sure footed and easily adjustable with light aids, he needed merely hints as guidance. He loved jumping but remained calm and regarded flying over fences as just another dressage exercise to be done with suppleness, grandeur and style. I felt very grown-up when riding him over a course of huge obstacles.

We had to walk our obstacle course before jumping them to make a plan as to how to approach and execute the jumps. After my walk, I had to report to Dr. Reznek my findings. On one occasion, I told him that I had a premonition that Gadara would crash into the tenth jump but all would be well and without injuries. Dr. Reznek said, "I will withdraw you from the class. I will not have you fall."

I pleaded not to do that because then there might be endless future "premonitions" crowding out my competition career. "Please do not believe my imagination." I pleaded.

Dr. Reznek saw my point of view and let me ride the course. At the tenth fence Gadara slipped from a mighty wide take-off point, and landed into the middle of the fence with me rolling off like a bowling ball. We both stood up, and Gadara behaving like an Edwardian gentleman eager to assist the needy, hastened to me, stood up four-square, waited for me to get back into the saddle and we continued the course accompanied by the sound of thunderous applause from the stands.

At the risk of seeming boastful, I confess that I never fell or was bucked off a horse but I did go down with my horses when they crashed into jumps four times, suffering no injuries. I consider this not merely "the luck of the dumb" but a special dispensation. Considering the immense number of jumps we took with hundreds of horses, four accidents seemed a very modest allotment.

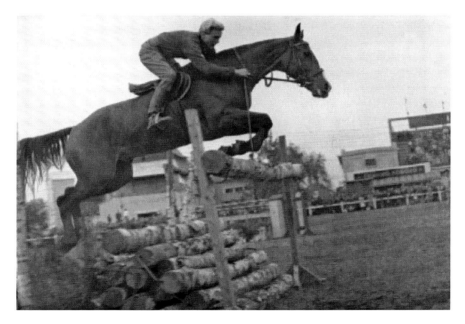

Gadara, secure and confident, competed on international jumping courses and also performed Grand Prix dressage.

Traditionally, the honor round of the five top-placing horses in a class was done in a handsome canter executed in a two-point seat. I always found an opportunity to show Gadara breaking from canter to passage to parade his ribbon, thus proving the "good boy" was highly schooled.

I inadvertently returned the generous favors of Bandi Bondor, lending his gorgeously trained horses to teach me. I had already moved to California when Bondor was given my horse, Kormend, schooled by me. Bondor rode him at Grand Prix at the Rome Olympics in 1960.

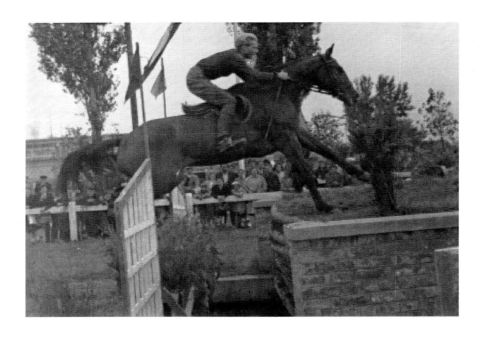

Gadara and I jumping up a bank over-water ditch.

REGOLY

Regoly was a mature bay stallion, nearly ruined and sullen by the time I got him. He had a low opinion of humanity and seemed bitter about people. Surely he had physical reasons for his peculiar way of jumping. He took all fences by ascending somewhat obliquely, darting above them to the left. One could lower the right rein and lead with it sideways to prevent the leftward jump but he took no advice. Regardless of my instructing him to take fences at ninety degree interception, he was taking them at his angle. Sometimes, without discernible cause, he got frantic, nostrils flaring, breathing hard when he was shown a fence. He must have remembered some ill-treatment in the past. At other times, especially when the fences were very high, he submitted to my adjustments on approach but knew that I was a helpless passenger over the fence, and consequently he jumped it at an angle, full period.

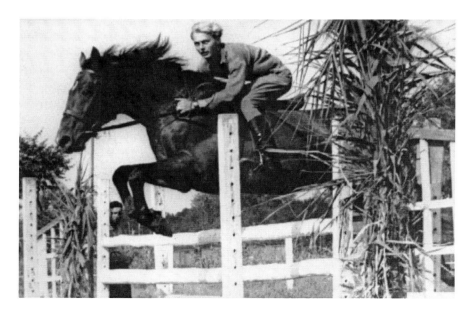

Regoly jumped fences by angling and bending to the left, not at the proper 90 degree intersection.

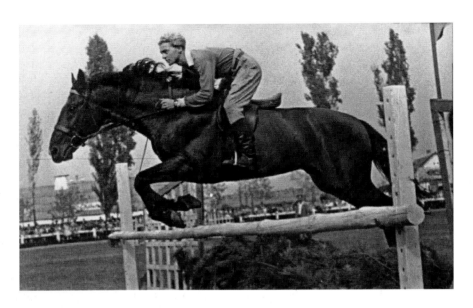

**Regoly was a difficult jumper.
I had to master his will tactfully.**

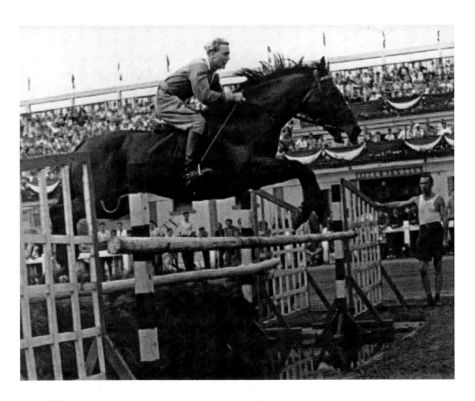

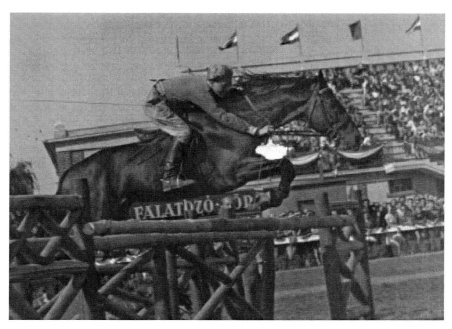

By lowering my right rein over fences I tried to induce his landing on the right lead to manage a right turn after a jump.

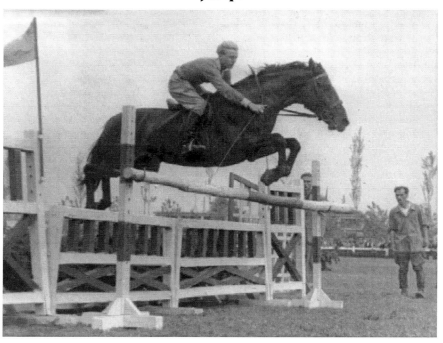

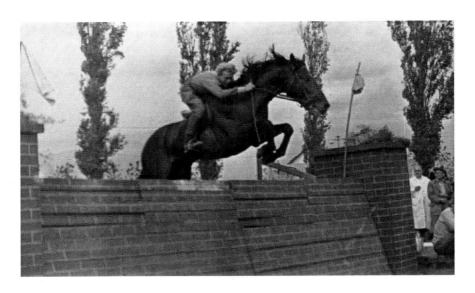

Regoly over a 160 cm. wall, winning, still turning his head left.

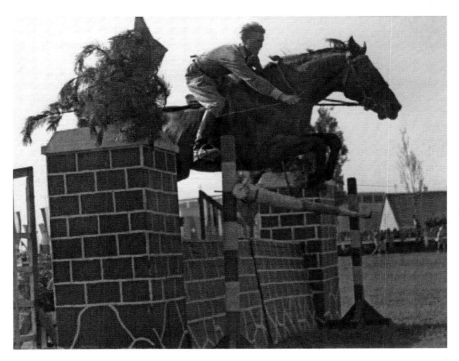

I felt perfect harmony with Regoly over fences.

70

Having finished a mighty difficult, and for him, a very high course (160 cm.) without any faults, he trotted out of the arena swinging his head low from side to side with a great sense of disapproval of what we just did. I kept petting and stroking his neck, hoping that he would think I agreed with him.

In dressage work, Regoly seemed bored and his natural gaits were meager. I was always encouraging suspension to make his strides more "dancing" and spare his badly configured body some jolts and trauma. All was in vain. His was very set in his ways. He showed little affection, and it was a red-letter day when he glanced at me in the morning as I said "Good morning" to my grooms. I felt practically privileged when he accepted a cube of sugar from me. Often he just dropped it on the ground and watched me bend over to retrieve it for him. He would look at me with critical sideways glances and then turn away joylessly. He pushed all my pity buttons.

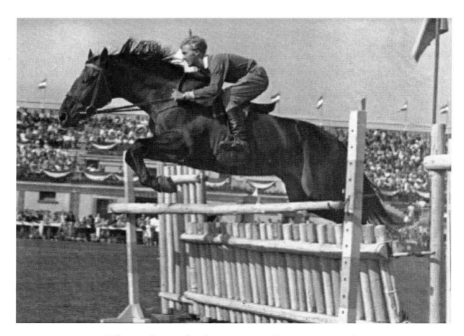

**I found my balance easily on Regoly
in front of a very large spectator attendance.**

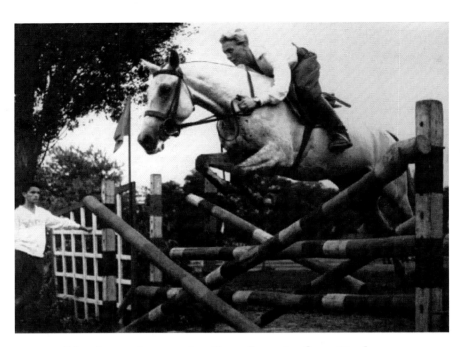

I had precise navigational control on Keringo.

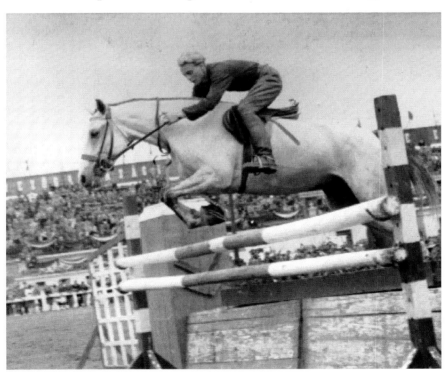

KERINGO

The name of this grey gelding means "waltz" in Hungarian. He was light, agile and good-looking. He could have made a handsome impression in any ballroom. He worked well and in good style on lower fences. For the short time I schooled him, he seemed like a pleasant riding horse without significant talent. He was eminently suitable for the riding pleasures of an amateur. It transpired that an Italian horse trader and owner of a riding school bought him to re-sell him for a profit. I am sure he succeeded. He was a sweet, attractive, and easy-to-ride horse. We were not allowed to talk with foreigners from the damned "Western Imperialist Camp," from which, ironically, this member of the Italian Communist Party emerged to seek his horse-

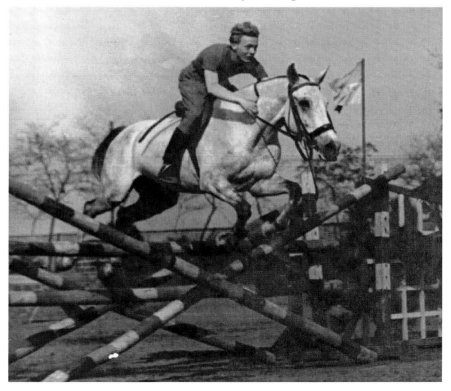

Keringo substituted talent for jumping with a calm nature, elegant style, exemplary suppleness and absolute obedience.

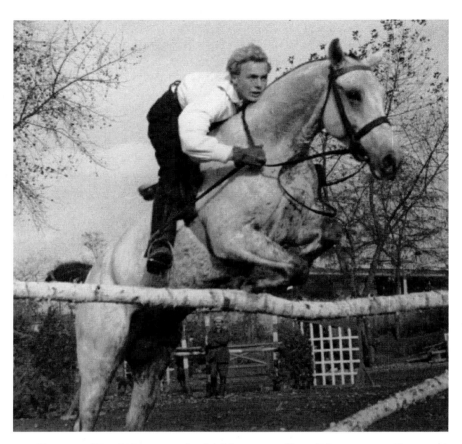

trading profits. We were forbidden to talk with one another, yet the irony was that just a few years earlier, this same gentleman had purchased a great many of my father's beef cattle and had shipped them back to Mussolini's Italy. At that time, he was a member of the Fascist Party. He was not received at our estate because he was a Fascist, but because he was buying farm products. Our family was strongly anti-Fascist and anti-Communist and suffered a great deal under both ideologies.

When I told my father about this Italian businessman's unexpected visit in Budapest and mentioned his current party affiliation, he said, "Italy is a small country, therefore they can spare only one set of fanatics that serve both socialist ideologies." When he was a Fascist guest, swanking-out in elegant comforts of our castle, I was just a child, and now he did not recognize me.

74

FOX TERRIER

Foxterrier was a well-routined jumper but he jumped in the wrong style, without a good "bascule." I was assigned to him to round his top line over the fences. He moved with a lumbering canter toward the fences making the earth rumble under his heavy feet. He was duty-bound, but not enthusiastic.

Hoping to preserve his energy, I gave him a very brief warm-up. He needed energy conservation more than repetition. I limbered him briefly by stretching his posture to gain the elevation of his reluctant back, and then jumped a few low fences. He knew his craft and grudgingly performed it. I trained him through spring and summer, competing with him a great deal before I managed to escape from Hungary. Therefore, I never really solved Foxterrier's problem of approaching fences hollow and jumping without a good bascule.

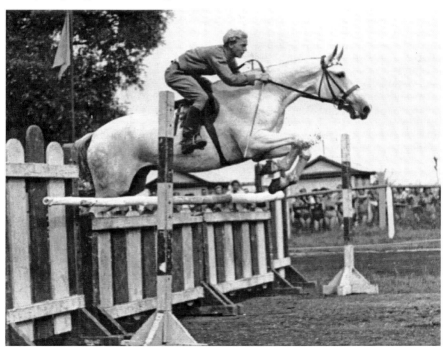

Fox Terrier was always jumping without properly raising and arching his back. My assignment was to changed that, but I escaped from Hungary before finishing my task.

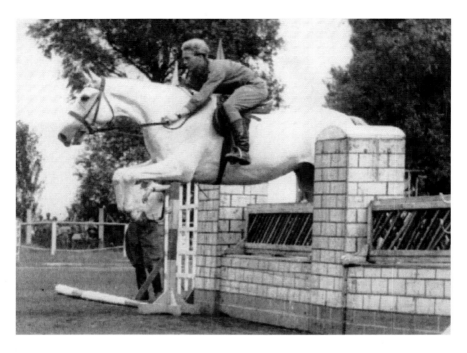

These images show me riding Fox Terrier for the first time in competition.

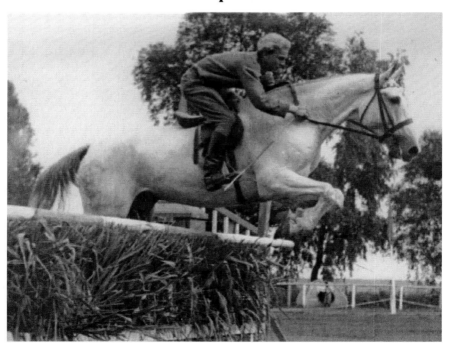

KOPE

A dark bay gelding named Kope was selected for me as a three-day-event prospect. He earned the experts' high regard because he was a Thoroughbred and an extraordinary mover. For eventing, we needed a fast horse with large strides to manage the demanding cross-country courses in good time. Good proportions along with floating, elastic strides were welcomed in anticipation of high dressage scores. Kope seemed to have all the necessary assets of a future three-day-event winner.

After a year of schooling, Kope refused to fulfill our expectations. He was certainly elegant about casually flipping poles off their pegs. He regarded fences as bowlers regard their pins. The more you topple, the better your score. On the cross-country course, fences are immobile and if the horse casually touches them all, he and his rider will not survive.

Kope remained a stadium fence demolition expert. He did not even seem to notice taking off all the top rails of the fences. He remained aloof and indifferent, such was his attitude

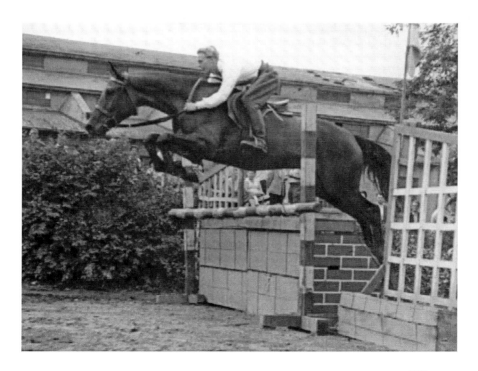

of *true elegance.*

I thought his problem might have been visual impairment but veterinary examination found nothing wrong with his sight. When he was dismissed from schooling, an illusion: hopes and dreams of Olympic glory, left with him.

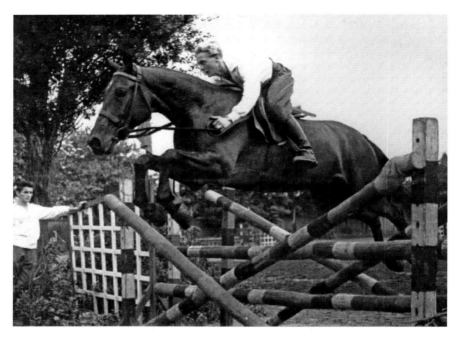

**I found harmony easily with the smooth elegance
of Kope's jumping style.**

NAPOLY

On a humid summer morning we set out single file through the main gate of the riding academy and turned right onto Kerepesi Avenue on our way out to the cross-country training grounds, and passed the racetrack, at Rakos Mezo. I was on one of my three-day event horses, a large-boned, flashy grey stallion with black mane and tail. His head sported a Roman profile common to the old Neapolitan bloodlines, yet his head was bony and dry with large, intelligent eyes adding to his nobility. His appearance illustrated the Baroque ideals. Napoly was the nickname I gave him. He had the majestic presence on which kings would be proud to enthrone themselves. He could have walked off a painting by Titian, Rubens or Velasquez but had he done so, he would have found me on his back instead of a king.

He had a willful, domineering character and I had to earn his respect slowly and dangerously. Eventually he condescended to work for me and appeared to enjoy his work. He certainly looked forward to seeing me. Every morning, upon my entering the stable, his massively deep and hugely loud trumpeting stallion-call greeted me. He did not nicker; he snorted, roared and bellowed. He also hurried sideways in his box to invite me in and I stepped on the high piled straw bed to give him his sugar cube, which he took delicately off my palm with quivering lips.

Most of us were riding stallions this particular morning and therefore proceeded single file with at least two horse distance between each of us to ensure some sense of safety. Stallions sometimes fought each other without warning. Once they did, the riders sitting on them would get bloodier and sustain more damage than the fighters beneath them. On days we worked geldings and mares we went out in pairs, although in silence, dictated by the protocol that forbade chatting while on horseback. Talking was a potentially hazardous inattention to the horse and the terrain, and therefore disrespectful to the horse. My teacher's admonition was "The horse is not a chair to just sit on idly. He is a partner you guide."

On the stallion-training day, we were walking in single file, and one could hear nothing but the clattering and slipping of hooves on the Macadam pavement. Soon we stepped onto the smooth, even more slippery asphalt surface of the avenue-wide bridge that spanned more than a dozen pairs of railways beneath it. The busy train traffic progressed in and out of the great Keleti Railway Terminal. On this average morning, trains rushed hastily under the bridge. Some were gliding express trains, while other laboring locomotives with hissing steam pulled unseemly freight at a snail's pace.

Having reached the middle of the span of the slippery bridge, my stallion suddenly reared up straight and tall on outstretched hind legs like a giant white candle. With the well-practiced instinct of a rider of many stallions, I hugged his neck and ducked my face sideways upon noticing his sudden ascent. I was hanging parallel with his strong body, also in a near vertical position, him hoisting me high with his massive neck. Being strong, he was "safe rearing," presenting no danger of falling backwards. His strong haunches and wide set hind legs could support his rearing for a long time. But his anger with the hissing locomotives and clattering rail wagons below knew no limit as he snorted and started to sway out of balance, repeatedly stepping backwards to regain his lost equilibrium. It never seemed to have occurred to him to put his front legs back on the bridge for better balance on four feet. As he swayed and backed towards the low concrete railing, he placed me just above the void that fell away a hundred meters below to the rails on which the killer trains rushed. I was dying a hundred deaths from the readily imagined falling of the horse backward upon me, crushing me below his mighty weight, to the visions of my arms failing to cling to his neck and I, free falling to my death. Images of a wretched survival of my fall flooded my head, followed by visions of being cut to pieces by the trains running over my limp and broken body.

Robbing me of my apocalyptic fantasies, my stallion dropped his forelegs down to the pavement. Propelled by his great excitement and gravity defying energy, he broke into a canter, bounding angrily in place on the slippery pavement where his shoes threw sparks.

The other riders came to a halt, turned around to witness my jeopardy and blanched as they anticipated my imminent demise. But smiles dawned on the flushed faces of my colleagues as they watched my big gray stallion canter in place, looking majestic with his huge, round neck set high and blowing heavily through his nose. I knew better than to smile because on safer ground he often used to bounce higher and kick out to discharge his excess energy. He might have started by cantering in place but then he would suddenly bounce higher, and explode into huge leaps. These eventualities were not welcome in my mind, for one of these leaps could have eased us over the low concrete railing and hurled both the magnificent stallion and his pale rider to a horrible death.

And so it transpired that we finally bounded in tiny canter strides off the bridge and proceeded to walk toward the cross-country course, as if nothing happened, in a calm single file. The anticipated jumping, climbing and sliding exercises in cross-country work now seemed child's play and I walked along, looking forward to them with a grin on my face.

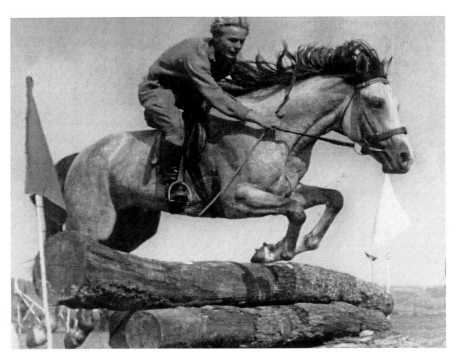

**Tyukod was so good looking
that I used to explain to friends, "He also jumps!"**

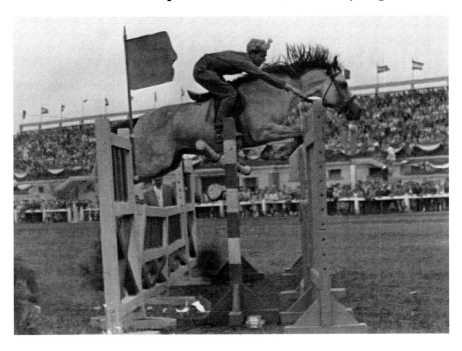

TYUKOD

Tyukod was a three-year-old stallion of very cheerful disposition when I got him. He was certified to breed for his tribe by the same name. Therefore, he also had a number after his name, informing us how many generations of his lineage were bred before him. He was a very springy and elastic mover. Sitting his trot was like riding a rather huge and fast passage. I felt like I was sitting on the apex of a hoop. He was gray with fabulous, good looks, which mattered to me. Call it vanity, but I like it because vain people are always clean. Tyukod also knew how to get attention just by being his lovable, good looking, intelligent, talented and splendid self.

As with all horses, Tyukod was required to do dressage, jumping and cross-country. He loved it all, but I was not deliriously happy with his cross-country work. When I showed Tyukod a jump of any height, he became enormously happy and

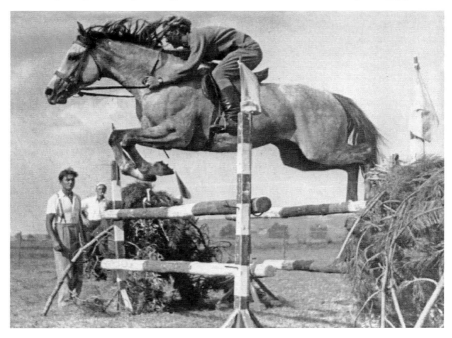

**My fabulously bouncing, buoyant
and gravity-defying Tyukod.**

started to "lançade" (lunges up and forward.) He approached the jump with incredibly high leaps, of which the smallest one was the last, the one that took us over the fence. Instead of allowing me to control his transportation by balance, rhythm, level of collection and a well-finessed take-off point to the fences; he ignored me as soon as I showed him a fence. He simply took over and with all his huge energy told me to buzz-off, hang on, pray and all would be well. He never took a pole but often came near to loosing me as he frolicked through the air like a dolphin in water. This kind of a partner out in wide-open spaces made tears flow horizontally out of the corners of my eyes. Fortunately, my wise coaches took him off the cross-country team. I was allowed to show him only in dressage and jumping events. He became one of three horses I ended up showing in jumping classes at the Grand Prix height of 160cm. His joy of jumping and his lofty, dancing trot strides were infectious signs of his optimism and he never failed to cheer me up even on my darkest days.

Because I adored him, Tyukod made me his fool and made my tutoring him about jumping nearly impossible. He let me know on every jumping lesson that he knew more about it than I would ever know; he was broadcasting his conceit with his entire body, "Let me do it! Let me do it alone!" And most of the time I had no other option.

The spectators' gallery loved him. Approaching all fences with his spectacular leaps, he usually got a standing ovation. I did not, however, get much respect for it from my coaches. They secretly thought that I provoked Tyukod's behavior because I enjoyed the thrill of it, and out of vanity, I did not want to "tone him down." My grooms referred to him as the "rubber ball."
The coaches' nickname for me was "the tranquilizer." I was respected for my successes in calming down the most nervous and high-strung horses. I rendered uncontrollable young stallions docile.

A day came when I was to compete in my home county of Tolna from which I had been exiled by the communist government. I needed special security police permission stamped into my internal passport in order to travel there. Curiously, through secret contacts and ministerial requisitions, permission was granted. In communism, of course, one has internal passports and travels at the whim of the police. The police could deny travel without stating why. External passports were unobtainable as people were locked up behind an iron curtain in a country that acted as a large prison.

When I competed in Tolna, people had to pretend not to recognize my well-known name. I was permitted to be there for only three days. On the last day of competition, there was a puissance class. In it, if the horse and rider clear a high fence, the judge permits them to continue jumping another round with a higher obstacle. Before I could jump each higher obstacle, I had to get my coach's permission by him signaling with his thumb up. If his stingy thumb were to turn downward, I was not permitted to approach the jump. There were only two riders left to attempt jumping higher when the judge rang the bell for me, inviting me to go for it. The jump was 186 cm. by then and my coach turned his thumb down. I, however, chose not to notice it, pretending that I had no time to glance at him because, after all, the judge summoned me by ringing his bell. I took off to the high jump on jubilant Tyukod bouncing, leaping, going crazy with happiness that he could jump something finally not beneath his dignity. Well, he cleared the fence at 186 cm. and my fellow competitor did not. And so it transpired that I won a puissance by clearing the highest fence that I had ever jumped. Tyukod was most satisfied, while the coach was murmuring threats.

KORMEND

Oh, my beautiful, gorgeous, generous and best friend, Kormend!

It must have been June when he was presented to me, because the soft, white cotton balls were floating from the cottonwood trees at the Tattersall. He gave me his attention for five years. He was a skinny, lanky, three-year-old red bay gelding and very friendly when we met. We fell into immediate mutual admiration upon meeting. He went straight for my straw-colored hair to taste it. Unfortunately the pulling and tasting of my hair went on for quite a while before Kormend lost his appetite for it.

All of my teachers agreed that Kormend was simply born for me, so he had to be assigned to me. I trained him to the

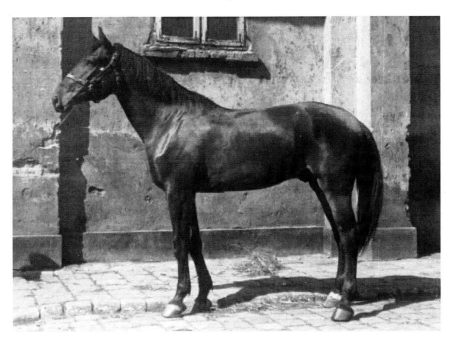

This is the way Kormend looked when I started with him. He went on to compete in the Rome Olympics 1960 in Grand Prix Dressage. His meager conformational resources were stunningly improved by his good will to always do our bidding.

86

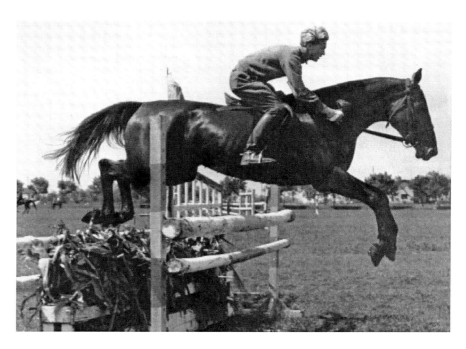

A record of our early competition career.

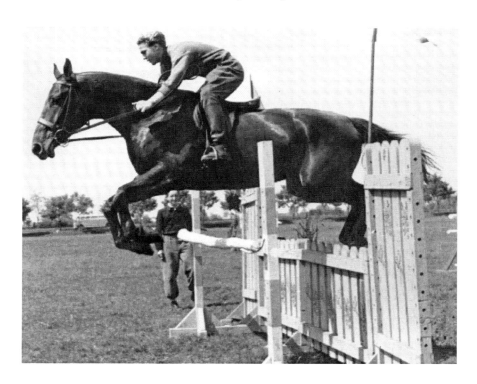

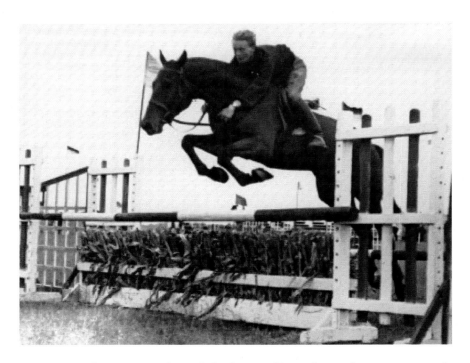

Kormend competed mainly in stadium jumping as part of his training for Olympic Three Day Eventing.

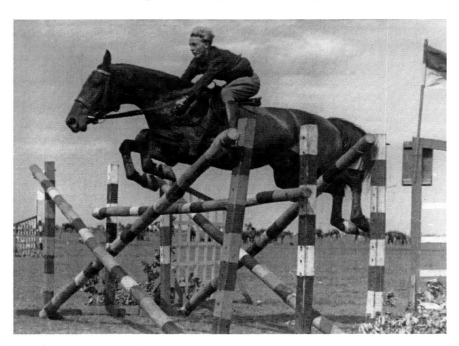

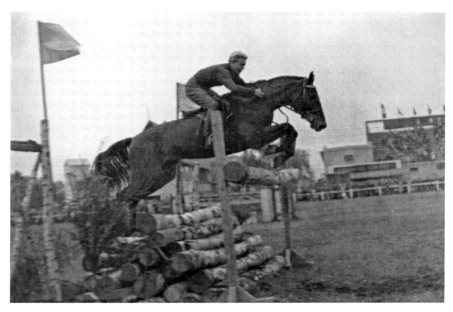

Kormend at the same competition that Gadara and I were also entered. Kormend placed first.

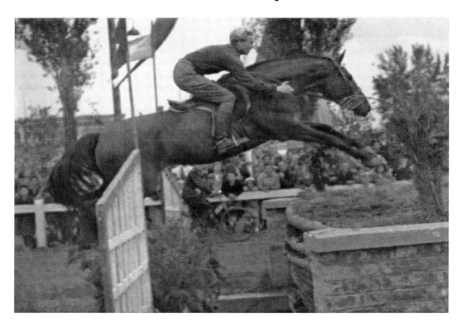

Once again, Kormend on the same jump, at the same competion, that Gadara and I were also entered.

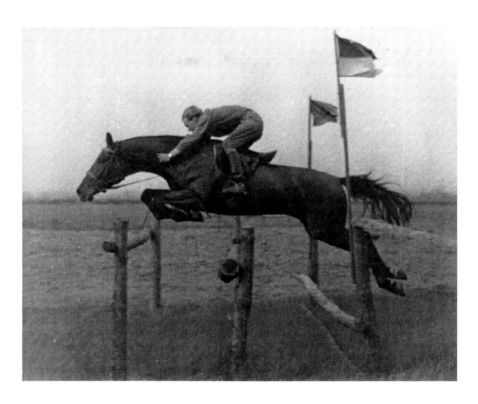

**Kormend in flight. What skills, what strength
from that 'backyard foal' that came to us!"**

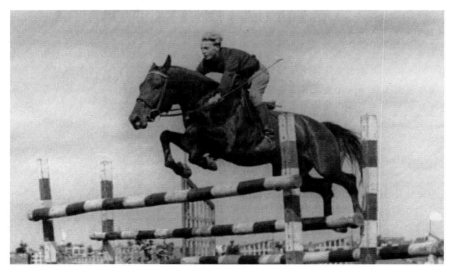

Kormend was safe, attentive and devoted to my commands.

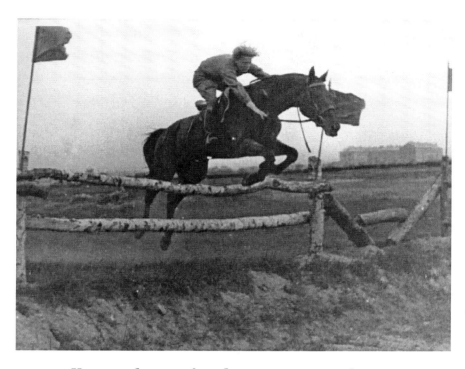

**Kormend executing the cross country jumps
on a full Olympic size course.**

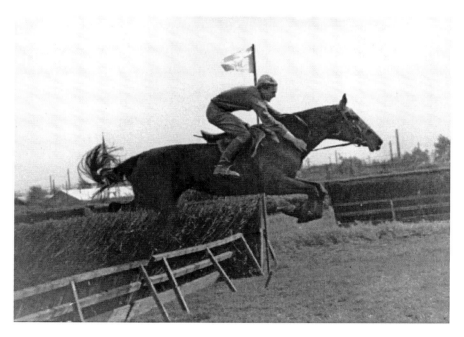

highest level in dressage. Everyone in our academy had to show his ability, knowledge, diligence and fitness by training completely green horses to the highest level allowed by their inborn talents. No one could graduate without having successfully schooled a horse to FEI level dressage. Schooling jumpers was naturally a faster process, but none of us were exempt from having to do both.

Years later, I was competing on Kormend in a high-level dressage test. I always forbade members of my family to attend my competitions and disturb my concentration. I had no time for society when my mind was on riding. When I rode well, whether in training or in competition, I was overcome by a meditative state from which I never wanted to be jolted. Perhaps my riding state of mind was akin to sleepwalking. If a sleepwalker is awakened, he falls from the roof on which he walked with certainty and security until jolted by another's call. My riding "death" also came when "awakened" from my meditative bubble in which there was only my horse and me with the world having receded.

In this particular dressage test, I was doing splendidly until, behind the judge at "C," a straw hat the size of a millstone appeared, festooned with silk flowers and fluttering ribbons. Under this inconspicuous accessory walked my mother with her long, elegant strides as resolute as a soldier's march and as graceful as a dancer's glide. The glorious hat swung its large brim in the rhythm of my mother's measured steps. Then my mother proceeded to become inconspicuous by settling directly behind the "C" judge, of course in full view to me. This broke my meditative bubble and jarred me back to the banality of daily life. My scores suddenly plummeted disastrously, proving that the judge actually was excellently discerning.

Kormend was my pride and joy because I groomed him into an outstanding athlete during five years of partnership. We bonded from the first day we met and he wanted to do everything for me. He was my "graduation gift." By the time I left him, in exchange for my life, he was the perfect Olympic-ready athlete that documented the correctness of our training. We had to groom to excellence the meager genetic resources allotted to our backyard peasant horses. To be sure, Kormend had assets too. He had a thoroughbred father that gave him courage, speed and stamina. He had the equine equivalent of Albert Einstein's brain and the patient attention of saints.

He was my best three-day-event horse and was prepared for Olympic courses. I will not detail our training protocol. He never stopped in front of a fence and never ran out either. His schooling was knowledgeable, systematic, gradual, and based on reward.

Finally, I rode him over a full Olympic level course. In those days, eventing was done on 25, 50, 75 or 100 percent courses. As the horses progressed in their athletic accomplishments, one advanced to compete on higher levels.

I hope that I still remember it correctly but by then my wonderful Kormend ate 34 pounds of oats every day. Work and food were knowledgeably administered and coordinated by professionals. Every Monday there was rest with a diarrheic diet to "cleanse" the horse's system. I know nothing about these things but want to report about the power of so much feeding of oats, giving my horse the enormous strength and endurance with which he carried me.

There was no such thing as a strong horse pulling your arms out of their sockets. Strength meant no disobedience and horses remained feather-light on the aids. I rode the dressage test on the first day of competition in a double bridle at the Prix St. Georges level. The horse was in self-carriage, absolutely light on the aids. The next day, we executed the 26 Kilometer 100% course with fixed jumps.

I was paired with a jockey on a racehorse to teach Kormend how to stroke the ground with stretched, elastic, ground-gaining strides. He loved to canter with his black racing companion and soon understood how to stay even with his challenger's strides. Kormend became clock-even in rhythm and vastly improved the length of his strides. During competing over fences on cross-country, his strides swallowed the kilometers effortlessly. Each jump seemed to have merely been fitted into one of those calm, even and generous strides. Kormend just flew over the cross-country course in absolutely even rhythm.

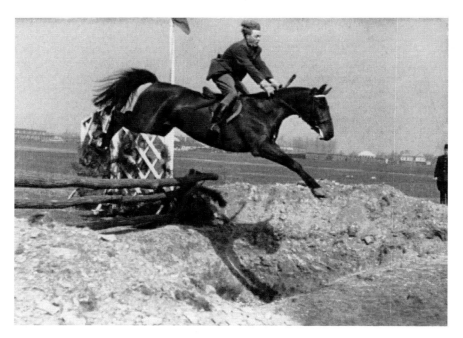

Here is the fourteen-foot wide ditch taken during the steeple chase.

In our dressage work we achieved a well-manufactured medium trot that floated with high cadence. It made our nine mile per hour trot requirement in the cross-country phase effortless.

Neither of us liked the steeplechase phase. At the fast gallop the horse assumes a very rapid four-beat canter, which the rider accommodates by floating above the saddle in a two-point seat, in short stirrups like a jockey. Without my seat telling the horse when to take off for the fence I trained my poor, tolerant Kormend to listen to my whip aids. I would gently stroke his side with the whip twice to warn him about the approaching take-off point, where I tapped him more strongly. Understanding these signals Kormend took the steeplechase jumps expertly and his confidence in me was surely deserving of a Nobel Prize. One of the steeplechase jumps was a fourteen foot wide ditch behind a slanted triple bar. The joke among my fellow competitors was that, "If you don't make it to the other side of the ditch but land in it, we will just shovel the dirt back to bury you."

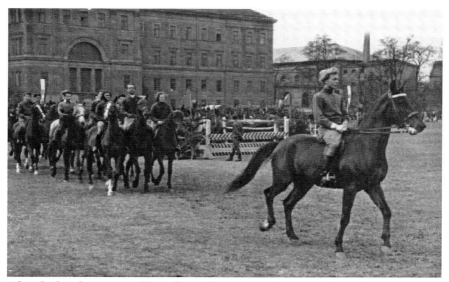

I had the honor of leading the squadrons of various teams preparing for the Stockholm Olympics. The gala took place in Kossuth Academy, Hungary's officers' school, in Budapest, 1956. We paraded in front of high-ranking officers of the Soviet Red Army. I blame them and their ear-shattering rendition of Soviet military marches, for Kormend not staying on my aids. By inverting his posture he apparently registered his disapproval of the proceedings.

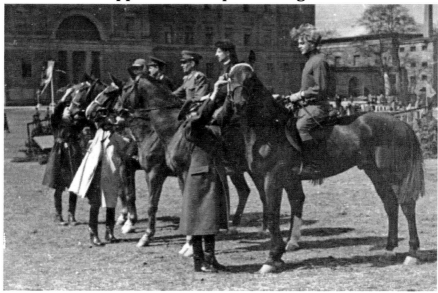

During the stamina-testing obstacle course I started to wilt and feel light-headed. Kormend sensed it and powered up hugely to inform me that he could carry even a wet rag over the course if only I could remain kind enough to show him which way to go. Not only did we survive the task, but we won the cross-country portion of the contest with no faults and in splendid time.

My poor horse was walked dry properly and when the veterinarian certified that all was well and his respirations were back to normal, he was lead back to his box, which was filled with fresh straw for him to sleep on. I was delivered there by a military jeep and found Kormend swanking-out on his royally supplied bed. By then, I was near collapsing because no one "walked me out" properly. I lay down in Kormend's box, my head against his stomach and we both fell asleep. I woke up when Kormend blew hot air in my face from his nose. I took his warning and jumped up before he did. With both of us standing and refreshed, the big day had ended.

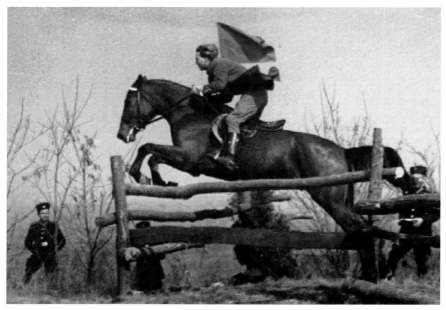

When I wilted in the saddle, he doubled his effort to console me. He had miraculously tucked away treasures of energy.

THE NAMELESS PROFESSORS

I have named the stars of my learning years but I must also pay tribute to the hundreds of others, the "extras." Without these "nameless" hundreds of horses, my education would have never been thorough. As Colonel Podhajsky so aptly reminds us: "Our horses are our teachers."

We can only know what we understand while riding each one of them. I had many horses to ride. I used to keep a log of these rides and in one year I rode over 200 different horses. We usually rode six horses each day.

The very basis of academic equitation was the belief that riders must learn to ride all horses – the species *equus* - to benefit any and all of them, and not just succeed at riding one "Dear Little Brownie." In the days of large cavalry regiments, riders had to ride a different horse each day to properly diversify their understanding of horses and hone their skills to ride them without harming them.

By the time I was at the academy, large cavalry units no longer existed. Therefore, the academy took on the assignment of preparing the young, three-year-old stallions for their *"korung."* For these stallion tests, young horses were to be tamed and trained to a certain standard of sophistication so that they could be tested and evaluated. We were assigned this task.

Even more important was the assignment, given to the riders in the academy, to prepare one hundred horses for the World Championship of Pentathlon in 1954. That event was assigned to Hungary to host as an honor for the Hungarians' winning the world championship of Pentathlon in Chile. In order to arrive at one hundred trained horses that would jump fences reliably under even weak riders we had to start training more. Not all candidates would stay healthy or become sufficiently skilled for the task. These horses had to be trained to carry any rider reliably over a cross-country jump course of about four hundred meters and jump about fifteen fences. The pentathlon participants were to pick the name of a horse from a wheel of fortune. Horse and rider never knew each other before the competition. The goal of training was to school a hundred horses to as even a level of performance as possible in order not to unfairly handicap any rider's performance with poorly prepared mounts. These horses had to do equally well in speed, endurance, tractability and jumping fences. The horses were expected to do well for any of the fifty or more competitors, which came with highly varied riding skills. These horses were not equal to our contemporary warm-bloods, but were gathered from peasant yards and state breeding farms.

We riders had to play musical chairs on two sets of horses. We had to ride a different horse every day by moving down one box in the stable to find the next unknown charger. The three year-old stallions were no joking matter. Neither was the program of building a hundred reliable cross-country competitors easy in a limited period of time. We learned to ride the species "horse" and not just our own horses. Later in my professional life, this education allowed me to ride any horse and improve them within minutes, to the great benefit of my students. Those training years earned me the later compliments that "He always makes it happen," or "It is like laying on of hands."

We were, indeed, diversified equestrians. We performed in dressage, jumping and on cross-country courses. We were lunged; we rode without stirrups, including on cross-country training sessions over jumps and up and down steep slides. Even the difficult and dangerous skills required for swimming with horses were acquired. We were required to learn herding of horses and distance riding. These were all considered essential skills and experiences for a well-rounded equestrian education.

Great teachers, their assistants, and even our peers tutored us, which diversified our skills but not our principles and methods. In upholding the classical training principles there was no tolerance for re-inventing equitation. One cannot make a first impression the second time.

In 1954 at the Pentatlon World Championships in Budapest, along with the stable staff, we were assigned to report to the Agricultural Exposition venue and hold horses there while they awaited their riders. We were warned by the secret police not to talk to any of the foreigners. I was told by an officer who, as

98

usual, knew more about me than I was expected to know about myself, "I know that you speak German. I am telling you that you are not to utter a word to any of the foreigners. They are not coming here to visit with you, understand? You are to pretend that you do not understand them and that you do not know any language by which you could communicate with them, understand? We will be watching." As if I didn't know that.

The competitors arrived in busses and cars, wearing riding attire, ready to compete. The Soviet team of four was noted because they were all doused with the same cologne, called Russian Leather. There used to be a popular scent for men in Hungary, called English Leather. Russian Leather had replaced the English Leather in the perfumery shops. This team's uniformity was again a sad example of dictatorship practiced to extreme. Where would one ever encounter an athletic team from a liberal western democracy using an identical scent? However, an uninformed Soviet KGB agent decided that polished grooming with a heady scent would impress the western visitors with Soviet indulgences in luxuries and displays of refinement. It was tyranny at its comedic best. One was flooded by compassion for the athletic peons so exploited by ignorance and vulgar taste. These fine athletes were practically embalmed by the scent they were surely not amused to wear.

The Austrian competitor, Herr Battig, approached me with confident strides as I held the horse with the number he pulled from the wheel of fortune. He presumed that I spoke German, which I did. With Viennese charm he addressed me with polite small talk and then inquired about the horse. Did I ride him? Was he good? Was he strong or light in contact? Did he need a lot of leg? Was he safe, obedient and fast? He asked many relevant questions to which I had the answers, but I was stifled by the orders of the secret police. My resolute silence and mask-like facial expression spoke volumes to Herr Battig, who finally said, "You are not allowed to speak to us, are you?"

I turned to the horse, pretending to check his girth and hid my face under the saddle's skirt to say quietly to him, "Ja, genau."

Two years later, I bumped into Herr Battig by chance, or by miracle, on the streets of Vienna. There I was a free man, certainly allowed to speak German in this most civilized country. I had successfully escaped the horrors of communist Hungary on November 22nd, 1956, breaking through the iron curtain. Now it was a bitterly cold, rapidly darkening December evening, whipped by cutting winds. As if we had a rendezvous we both wanted to keep, Herr Battig and I darted into the Café Havelka. We competed to speak, anxiously and rapidly to pour out the dammed-up tumult of memories. We sat in the glowing warmth of Havelka for a long time, and never ran out of the many things two utter strangers must tell each other. Yet, we had only seen each other for a few minutes two years earlier when I handed him his horse.

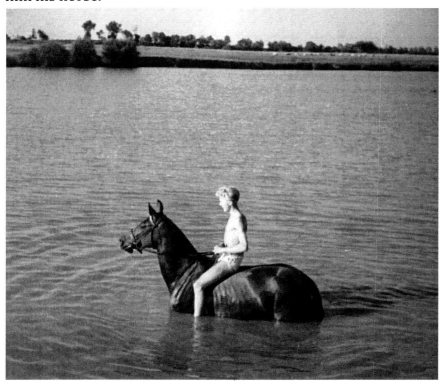

The author ready to swim Sator across and the wide but placid Koros River and back. A very dangerous undertaking that only riders with specific expertise should ever attempt.

DISTANCE RIDING ASSIGNMENTS

Distance riding and herding horses, called *Csikos* in Hungarian, were required diversifications of riding experiences. The longest distance ride I took was from Budapest to Siofok on the northern shores of Lake Balaton. A three day journey due to the ample rest periods for the horses – not for the riders. We had a wonderful time. One peculiar pleasure the communist regime inadvertently provided to us was setting the clock back to the nineteenth century. We encountered no motorized traffic, no one seemed to be working the vast fields, and divine silence everywhere. No one dared to chatter loudly or laugh conspicuously with uncontrollable screams and hooting. As the saying went, "We learned to move close to the wall and to live in the shadows." Calling attention to oneself, being conspicuous with too much visibility, invited danger.

Sixteen riders prepared the horses in the pre-dawn, opaque summer night. We set out at dawn and rode in the cool morning when the earth, the grasses and the crops were scented and shimmering with dew-flooded beads. In the silence, the sneezing of horses was muffled; quiet riders listened to the various melodies of competing songbirds. As the sun made an oversized, orange appearance, skylark songs followed us through the ripening wheat fields.

We were welcomed into the quiet, poverty-stricken peasant courtyards. When the heat became stifling, we unsaddled, the air dense with the buzzing and snapping sounds of bugs. The riders leaned on trees, sheds and arcades and idled in silent contemplation, chewing on the sweet ends of young grasses. The enchantment of that journey came from its re-enactment of life in the nineteenth century. I often felt homesick for the civilized culture of the past.

Another time, I rode with my groom, Imi, from Budapest to legendary Orkeny the former home of the old riding academy. By then, it was defunct; we had to deliver two horses and bring two others back. Our assignment served the task of horse transportation and doubled as an educational experience in distance riding. We did the return trip on the same day. Fortunately, we were young and immune to pain. Surely Napoleon's soldiers spent longer days in their saddles on their march from Paris to Moscow.

HORSE HERDING DUTIES

When we were assigned to be horse-herds we were overjoyed because we were sent to Bakonypoloske, a remote corner of the earth in a picturesque and pastoral mountain setting every bit as beautiful as a Le Brun landscape painting. It was formerly a famous Thoroughbred stud farm owned by a Czech Count, who by then had been "liberated" from it by the communists. Now, the little chateau with its superb neoclassical architecture was derogated to be a tractor station, tractors being the pride and joy of communist propaganda. We were not to notice that there were no functioning tractors anywhere on this collective farm. When we arrived, they cooked inedible meals in the chateau's kitchen for the members of the collective farm, and us, the uninvited guests. We ate our supper al fresco in the remains of the once beautiful park. After the first evening meal all four of us suffered from food poisoning and felt deathly sick during the sleepless night and for almost the entire day following it. We tried to find out which one of the many unappetizing things they fed us caused our misfortune but the only answer we received was that for dinner "We ate the bull."

When we recovered, our work was explained to us. It started at 4 AM. The mares with their young foals were to be herded out to drink and graze before the heat of the day. The short summer nights were pale and warm. The sun rose early and the air became heavy and hot. Each of us was assigned to one of the employees, all young peasant boys, and we went out in pairs with a reasonable sized herd. I was put under the wing of a very handsome peasant boy that conversed only about his envy of our privileged life in Budapest, where he had never been. Just by having come from the capital, I received his unqualified admiration. He even envied his own imagination of a life in Budapest.

102

He presented me to an old, boney, dignified black mare, faded by months of sun bleaching. When I was lead up to her, she was standing motionless as if she were to be lead to her crucifixion. The so-called saddle handed to me was a lemon-yellow piece of felt, cut to resemble the shape of a real saddle but had neither frame nor girth. It did have two stirrups, however, with the stirrup leathers cleverly stitched to the felt pad, their lengths non-adjustable. "One size fits all" had already been adapted as a socialist motto. Obviously there were no individual riders, only the "community" of riders.

I wondered how one would get on the boney mare without a mounting block, a groom's assistance, a pair of proper stirrups or even a saddle secured by a girth. My new mentor was very encouraging by suggesting, "Just jump up, then find the saddle and sit on it because her spine sticks out."

We let our herd out of the enclosure and the horses all started to run and frolic in the vapory air. My mare volunteered to canter on the left lead while the friskier young mare carried my colleague on the right lead. The herd volunteered to do everything without our tutoring and I was amazed at how well they behaved. First they stopped to drink at the little brook that meandered around, very suitable for a conventional landscape painting. Then the herd ran a little while and when they arrived in a large meadow, they filled it up by spreading out more thinly to graze. A dense forest of ancient oaks, also properly arranged for framing the gorgeous meadow, was suitable for an ideal landscape painting.

As the mares spread around the large meadow, the sun rose as if on cue and my mare stood up squarely. She lifted her boney head skyward on her razor-blade thin neck, kept it horizontal to the ground, and closed her eyes pretending to be sunbathing somewhere in the Caribbean. I sat prudently on her yellow felt-covered, skinny spine and awaited my fate. There was no wait long enough to engender daydreaming. From a standstill, sunbathing posture, the mare transformed herself into a race horse bursting out of a starting gate, determined to win the race. Off we went, still together. I grasped a large tuft of mane that stood straight up in front of her withers. I understood why hairs of her mane remained stubbornly vertical. Surely, others had hung on to them all day in anticipation of the re-enactment of a departure from the starting gate.

The mare, it turned out, was on an errand, and not at the races. With seemingly closed eyes, she spotted some vagrant foals drifting away from their mothers, or horror of horrors, away from the herd toward the darkness of the oak forest. Well, duty called and the mare needed no prompting. She galloped with lightning speed to catch the foals and herd them back to their dams. This she did with rapid shifts of directions and tight turns into which she leaned like a speeding motorcycle in a curve. I lived through some five minutes of this without falling off, my hair flying vertically, the mare's mane clenched in my fists.

The peasant lad thought it amusing and commented with discernible bitterness, "You did not fall off." After an hour or so, and with several similar repeated episodes, he finally approved by noting, "You got balance."

And I was thinking, yes, eighteen months of lunging will do that.

CHAPTER 6

ANECDOTES

When you are "building socialism" you have inevitable shortages. No one bothers to explain what socialism looks like when it is finally built. One is just constantly whipped to build it without flagging enthusiasm. There is no way one can list all the things that are not available. It is easier to mention the few things that might be available. The realistic joke went like this: After your days were spent at "socialist labor," you went to queue up and stand in line for the necessities of life. Almost three hours later you got to the window where goods were dispensed and said, "May I have my bread allotment?"

To which the clerk replied, "If you want to stand in line where they are out of bread, you must go over to the line on the right. Here you are in the line where we ran out of lard." For telling this and hundreds of other jokes, one could get a sentence of ten years of hard labor. These labor camps were called "re-education camps" because in Communism everybody is a "beneficiary" of a free education.

Not long before my father was condemned to exile and taken away to a concentration camp in June 1951, I accompanied him to a nearby jewelry shop. He was collecting his Breitling stopwatch that was being repaired. The store attendant, masquerading as the jeweler, was a secret police career officer. While we were in the store, a tiny, elderly, emaciated lady entered and put a diamond brooch in a blue silk box in front of the attendant and asked "How much could you give me for this?"

To which the attendant extended his ridiculous offer of a pittance. Glass jewelry could have fetched more. The aristocratic lady tried for a better price by attempting to break the attendant's unbreakable heart. "This is my last good piece and I have nothing to eat anymore."

The clerk repeated his earlier, miserable offer. Then, the lady suddenly brightened up as a shining hope of an idea occurred to her and asked the clerk, "What do you think I could get if I sold it on the black market?"

And to this, the briefly honest secret policeman said with a smirk, "Oh, about ten years of hard labor."

We cast our eyes down to shield all emotion while the frail lady left with her little blue box.

Basically, food was scarce. Choices were limited. The quality of food was poor and the quantity allowed per person was restricted. If the authorities spotted your anti-social behavior of somehow getting more food than they thought you ought to have, you could have been imprisoned with the charge of being a "hoarder." In short, socialism was not a "decadent consumer society." Therefore, it transpired that we, having been selected for international riding and prepared to compete in the Olympics, became privileged by receiving an extra stipend (some money) to buy expensive food, such as meat. We even received coupons that entitled us to visit special stores that served only the Communist elite and foreigners. As would be expected and becoming of all good "classless societies" with the appropriate "social justice," the police prevented average citizens from stepping into privileged shops, exclusive buildings, and even some streets. We were always hungry, not starving, but malnourished. It was in these times that I realized I would eat anything that did not eat me. Our dietary needs were: food!

In totalitarian governments, state control is total, hence the name. Sportsmen like us needed state control not merely of sexual activity but even of hormonal desires! Therefore, we were required to drink a tea made of rose hips. The authorities believed that it made men impotent for a while. Physicians did not subscribe to this theory, but they were not consulted. The "Party Line" never relied on expert opinion or scientific validation. Experts just believed that rose-hip tea had some vitamin C in it and is rather benevolent. We drank the tea and, being a teenager, I must report that it failed in its officially designated function.

THE REMARKABLE PEOPLE
AROUND ME

I had a great aunt that used to say, when describing others, "Nice people, but not our circle." During my four years of academic training many nice people were around me and many of them were certainly not part of our circle. Come to think of it, not everyone was nice. When someone was undeservedly designated as "nice," my snide remark was "Everyone is nice that does not steal a locomotive in broad daylight." That kind of commentary earned me the reputation of being cynical.

I accepted the pleasure of knowing interesting people due to my equestrian schooling. These remembrances are vehicles of paying tribute to, and expressing gratitude for the interesting people I knew. All my life, I was privileged by my friendships and fascinated by my acquaintances.

PISTA HEGEDUS

Pista Hegedus was a famously beautiful man. His figure, designated by Hungarian exaggeration, was considered to be the most perfect male image. He was a modern-day Adonis. His image as the ideal nude athlete was on the Twenty Forint bill of Hungarian currency. Rumor had it that the French Academy

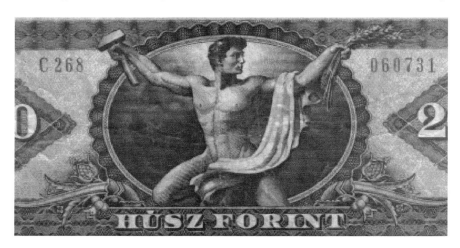

of Sciences had already reserved his future corpse for their collection and scientific studies. I watched him ride as often as I could. He rode mostly indoors and in solitude on a very beautiful horse. The aesthetics of these experiences were superb and I was glad to realize that I was his only spectator on a daily basis for a long time. I was in awe of him, an aesthetic monument to manly beauty, and he was aware of that, as he was not stupid. My mother's admonition came to mind: "Great beauty has its obligation. For the very beautiful can as easily hurt the feelings of those ignored, as can enchant those to whom he pays attention."

When I was requisitioned for the filming of "Rakoczi's Lieutenant" at Lillafured, he was also there, being used as an officer and a rider. Most everybody called him by the strange nickname of "Fityula." I don't even know what that stands for. We became friends, but my behavior changed in his presence because I wanted to impress him. I became self-conscious. I remained uncharacteristically silent, when in his company. The Latin admonition *"Si tacuisses philosophus mansisses"* [Had you remained silent, you would have remained a philosopher] was ringing in my ears. I wanted to appear sophisticated. Yet surely silence was not my best calling card at the time.

Two years later Pista married a beautiful brunette. It was an enhancement of his great beauty to be connected with that of another. Just as before he and his gorgeous horse, now it was he and his gorgeous wife.

Soon after his wedding, during the Hungarian uprising, he was mowed down by Soviet machine gun fire as he walked among an unarmed throng on his way home. I was told by someone who claimed to have witnessed it that Pista was actually cut in half by the bullets.

DR. FERENC VOLGYESI

Dr. Volgyesi was allowed to pursue his passion for dressage riding because he was an internationally known psychiatrist and author. He was well-known abroad and even travelled in the United States before the war. Therefore, he was allowed the meager privileges afforded to few select citizens by the Communist regime. The regime was eager to advertise civilized well-being in the lifestyle of those that were "visible" to the West. Everyone was evaluated by their value to the regime and treated by the state accordingly.

Dr. Volgyesi was a very good rider because he understood horses and was devoted to their wellbeing. He was very smart, well-educated, and a cultured connoisseur of the arts with many published scientific writings. He had a most interesting face, suitable to be worn by Ancient Romans on coins or by the Renaissance poet, Ludovico Ariosto (as depicted by Titian) or even by Lorenzo de Medici (The Magnificent.). He had beautiful, richly wavy, graying black hair. With his deportment he could have starred in a film as a 19th Century diplomat.

His Grand Prix trained mare was a delicate-looking gray. Once, while this mare was shipped by freight train to a country town for competitions, I travelled with her along with some grooms in the same proverbial "cattle car." When the train moved, the mare started to trot in place, as if on a treadmill, and performed the piaffe during the entire trip. It was an exhausting experience for all of us, the difference being that we kept her cool by washing her down repeatedly during the trip. The mare was never the worse for her hysterical travel excitements and casually won her competition classes.

Dr. Volgyesi lived with his twenty-year old son, Sandor, who was a wrestler. He had angelic blue eyes with angelic expressions, highly unbecoming to the image of a fierce fighter. Sandor looked as if he were a confiscated angel-image from a Renaissance painting. During my last two years in the academy, they both became my friends and invited me to dinner every Tuesday night. I was always hungry and they ate better and more privileged food than I usually did. I would never forget my first visit to these fabulous Tuesday evening meals.

The son, Sandor, opened the door. Inside the dark entrance hall one could see many doors leading to several different rooms, each of which was occupied by different strangers in this "community apartment." Similarly, where my grandmother lived alone, and in which then I lived, was also subdivided to house four different families. This was the new norm of life with rampant scarcity.

I was guided in the twilight of the crowded entrance hall, straight to the door opposite the entrance. There I was ushered into a cavernous room, suitable to be the Grand Salon of a palatial mansion. The lofty ceiling was frescoed and the walls were hung by apple-green silk. The evening light seeped in through three virtually floor-to-ceiling French doors that lead to balconies in the Parisian style. As if by magic, I was once again in the familiar space of a grand room suitable for a mansion. A strange small space, what may have been a butler's pantry, was behind a secret door camouflaged by the green silk of the walls. Then, that was used as a bedchamber, heavily draped and as romantic in mood as any would be in Second Empire Paris.

By now, I felt as if I were in a privileged, royal presence and yet the great pleasures were yet to come. The walls were crowded, and I mean from ceiling to floor like in Florence's Palazzo Pitti, by the greatest paintings of the masters of the Golden Age of Hungarian paintings. Between 1815 and 1945 Hungary was second only to France in master-painters. All the works on these walls were by the greatest names among the finest masters of Hungarian painting. I recognized almost every one from the pages of art books. But now I was standing in front of them, talking about them, dreaming about them, and an hour later eating supper in their company by candle light. As we visited these masterpieces, tightly arranged on the walls, Dr. Volgyesi mentioned that he had many more canvasses in secret storage. I teased him by saying, "I am not sure that you like paintings but I am convinced that you do not like the sight of walls." I found myself in an oasis of beauty and culture at a time of general deprivation and brutality.

During the dinner there was only candlelight in this grand room. A housekeeper prepared the delicious meal and served it in silence. Her white apron and silence told me that she always served and her toothless, narrow lips showed off her dignified poverty. There were candles everywhere: in French ormolu candelabras, in cut crystal candelabras, and in silver candlesticks

110

engraved with nine-spiked crowns on them. Everything flickered and quivered on the walls from the liquid lights of dozens of blazing candles. On the sideboard, tumbling out of an enormous bronze vase, were outsized white and purple peonies. We became inhabitants of a great canvas, which could have been painted by Vuillard. We had much to say and we said it quietly in deep tones as the evening wore long and the candles melted into oozing puddles and drooped into long drops while their wicks burned to their bases.

I was fed festive food at these special dinners. But the great gift to my life was being in the company of a cultured father and an enlightened son. A comfort of the spirit overcame me when in the company of these like-minded people and kept me in a mood as if bewitched and transported to a magical world. During these evenings everything outside this room and everyone other than these two men suddenly seemed alien, inexplicable, unnecessary, and unwanted.

PROFESSOR ROSENBERG

I am declining the professor's real name. He was a famous Jewish scholar, and expert on the Middle East. He specialized on Islam and the Arab cultures and he used to live in Syria, Lebanon, and Egypt while he travelled widely. He survived the National Socialists simply because he was unavailable to be murdered as he absented himself abroad in territories controlled by the Allies during the war. The Soviets had many designs on the Middle East, animated by ambitions to shut down the oil supplies to industrialized nations, thereby choking them. The professor was viewed and treated by the Communists as a great asset.

He was a passionate rider, and around horses exhibited very British manners. These were augmented and accompanied by magnificent riding boots from London and other fineries of distinguished British origins. He was short and chunky but looked good on his very tall, slender, grey gelding. He trained it very well. Knowledge had seeped into him during his life in the Middle East. I watched him "assemble" his gelding at the halt, with great generosity of time allotted to this artistry. By the time he looked satisfied with the horse's "assemble" he could cajole him into a spectacular Piaffe right on the spot.

The professor's life seemed like a fairy tale. He was not only allowed, he was ordered to travel out of Hungary, cross the iron curtain and do whatever he was ordered to do at the targeted Mid-Eastern region. He also came back. He must have been so "compromised" by the regime that he would rather not defect.

Once I asked him after his return from one of his "official missions" to the Middle East, "Where do you like it better? Here in Hungary or over there in Lebanon?"

He turned to look behind his shoulder just to be sure that no one was listening, and answered quietly, "I like it best during transit!"

I understood his witty message and thought that if an informer had heard that, he would also get a sentence for ten years of corrective labor. I somehow admired this political, scholarly and secretive vagabond. And I did not mind watching his mastery of riding piaffe either.

ERDODY

It was only in hind-sight that I realized the obvious, that Erdody was an informant. A strange expression it was, but secret police agents were assigned to observe and report on us and we talked about them as having been built on top of us. I still cannot fathom how many of us were placed under Erdody's supervision. He was unusually good at hiding his real identity and function. In fact, I was unaware of his assignment to inform on me until the very end of it. I realized his years of "friendship" with me were sinister and politically assigned. His "job" of ensnaring me, however, led him eventually to feel some genuine kindness and affection toward me. I realized his true identity only few months prior to my fleeing Hungary. I feel compelled to obscure his identity. The choice of his name by me is arbitrary. It is, however, imitating the secret police tradition of giving their agents new names that sounded like "good old Hungarian names of better families." I try to follow this prescription in my writings and hide the real identities of these people, the bearers of "good old Hungarian names of better families."

Erdody was simply permitted to ride with the students of the Academy and receive instruction with the members of the Olympic Teams, which were being prepared for Stockholm. Everything was commanded "from above" and such commands could not be questioned. He had to be accepted as he worked for the Ministry of Agriculture. I think now that I may have been the only person so naïve as to accept everybody and everything at face value. I forgive myself on account of my youth. Perhaps all others around me were wise to his identity and function. But I do not even now recall the usual secretive winks and nods we used to signal each other in order to broadcast such sinister dangers.

Erdody befriended me by talking intelligently about riding and also in a sly way about "the good old days." He was siphoning information from me and monitoring my emotional responses. I found him always next to me, acting like my "big brother." My first two years of schooling were done at the Tattersall. However, the last two, including training toward the Stockholm Olympics, were done in the Kossuth Akademia, which used to be the famous Ludovica, Hungary's equivalent of West Point. I did not read any danger sign into Erdody being also transferred with us to the very exclusive, strictly forbidden territory of Kossuth Akademia.

He asked me to join him and his wife, a sullen and uneasy woman of great intelligence, in excursions to the very few nightclubs that remained maintained mostly for spying on foreigners and diplomats that gathered in them. I noted one suspicious incident at a time when he invited me to see a movie. At the entrance of the theater, a young man lifted his dark green, gorgeous Austrian hat to greet Erdody with some formality and deference. A lady friend, much concerned with my welfare, had already pointed out this young man to me with the succinct comment, "He is dangerous." I never asked Erdody who that young man was and how it was that he knew him, pretending that I did not notice the incident. I was by then well-aware of the dangers in revealing to agents any suspicions by asking them questions. Erdody encouraged social contact with me beyond camaraderie in the riding academy. Sometimes he managed to time his tram rides to Kossuth Academy to coincide with mine.

Later, during the hazardous days of the Hungarian uprising he asked me to let him accompany me home because he lived nearby and he thought he could perhaps protect me. There was still a great deal of fighting in the capital. We dodged bullets daily. There were huge throngs of humanity in the avenues and boulevards because of the general strike that stopped all public transportation. Erdody and I were walking for a long while from Keleti railway terminal down on Rakoczi Avenue and arrived at its intersection with the Grand Boulevard. Scattered in chunks and splinters were the last remains of the immense bronze statue of the hated tyrant, Stalin, being hacked apart for bits of souvenirs. At the moment we stepped into that intersection, a barrage of machine gun fire was unleashed on us from rooftops and upper floors of the surrounding buildings, as if waiting just for our arrival. The unarmed crowd broke into a howl–the kind that curdles the blood in one's veins–and started to stampede. The flood of bullets herded the crowd essentially in one direction. The machine gun bullets carved arcs into the pavement, cut grooves into the asphalt and were accompanied by a din of exotic clattering sounds. Erdody grabbed my arm with great strength, determined not to lose me in the tumult.

He dragged me in a fast run as we watched people flying around from impact, collapsing, screaming, crawling in blood, running over the fallen living and stampeding over the moaning dying. I watched in disbelief a severed head rolling in front of me as if I were following a football, trying to catch up to it. In this head, open eyes rolled in a circle. Then, suddenly I could not see and hear. When I became conscious and sensible, I was sitting next to Erdody on a wooden crate. He was holding me up by hugging my shoulders as I leaned against him. I felt no strength in my lower back and felt too weak to hold myself upright. We were in the storage basement of the "Kozert" grocery store on the very corner of this deadly intersection. Outside there was still gunfire, gradually becoming sparse. We sat there in silence

114

with another dozen or so pale people staring at us.

I cannot remember when Erdody lead me out of the hiding place and we started to walk–by now in dusk–on Dohany Street toward home. There was a problem. I could not speak. I wanted very much to thank Erdody or make some pleasant gesture, but I could not. I lost my ability to speak, or sob or make any sound. My brain's commands were dishonored by my voice. Erdody led me by the arm and looked at me from high above, as he was much taller. He kept saying, "It's all right. You are very well. You are not wounded. You behaved very bravely." Then, at the door of our flat, he tipped his hat to my mother, whispered something directly to her ear and helped me into bed. Then, I heard vaguely that he talked to mother quietly.

By the time this gesture of kindness, prompted by his genuine fondness for me transpired, I knew the real identity and mission of Erdody. Based on merit, the Council of Coaches submitted the names of twelve riders deemed ready and deserving to compete at the Stockholm Olympics. I was among them. We were sworn to loyalty at the usual pompous ceremony in the Katona Jozsef Theater. We were warned–as if we did not already know–that our entire family would be jeopardized or doomed if we were to defect once outside the iron curtain. As usual, merit was replaced by political expedience. Only four of the twelve riders were granted exit visas and a passport, while the rest of us were judged "politically unreliable" by the secret police. I think that Erdody was not consulted and was not needed to veto my exit visa. Obviously, the communist secret police would never allow the likes of me to cross to the other side of the iron curtain.

Three months after the denial to participate in the Stockholm Olympics, in November of 1956, I escaped to freedom under horrendously hazardous circumstances. Thereby answering the cynical question of people taking liberty for granted, "Is it better dead than Red?" – Yes.

A few months later, I moved to Big Sur, California and I received my mother's letter reporting that Erdody "committed suicide" by falling from the fourth floor of the inner balcony of his apartment building. We knew that these "suicides" were often the result of four secret police thugs throwing a desperately struggling victim off the upper floors of buildings where they had been deliberately assigned their living spaces on high floors. I wondered, and still do to this day, whether his death was really a suicide. Could it have been prompted by fear of torture and punishment for "having lost" us, his wards when we successfully escaped? Or, was he actually thrown to his "suicide" by secret police thugs?

My young cousin was murdered by the secret police exactly in this manner in on February 18th, 1976. He was assigned an apartment on the fifth floor of a building and forced by blackmail to marry an "assigned wife" with a rank in the secret police. My cousin's wife "forgot" to lock the front door and took a long bath during which four strong thugs arrived and entered the apartment. According to witnesses, a long struggle commenced as my slender cousin fought for his life the four hefty men. They dragged him to the balcony over the inner courtyard and threw him over the rail to fall five stories to the tiled courtyard. There he died after three hours of agony at 11:30 PM while the police stood guard to prevent an ambulance or anyone else from approaching him. Such things "had no witnesses" and people "melted into the walls," pretending not to have heard or seen anything. One always had to pretend never to have witnessed secret police actions.

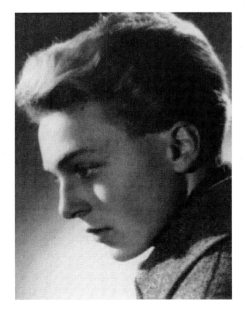

The author at the end of his academic schooling and only two months before escaping from Hungary.

CHAPTER 7

TRAGEDIES

On the 4th of November 1956 I woke up around 3:00 AM to the sounds of heavy artillery fire, bazookas and aerial bombardment. These were now familiar sounds, but this day they were impacting very near and the house shook and shuddered. I ran to my mother's room to tell her loudly in an irritable voice, "Let's go to the air raid shelter, we are under attack."

My mother woke not from the cannonade and bombardment but from my irritable mood and asked calmly, "What time is it?"

"Does it really matter? Can't you hear what is going on? And by the way it is three a.m." I yelled with agitation.

Then she turned toward the wall on which hung gorgeous Swiss embroidery from the fourteenth Century, and quietly said, "I sleep until eight. Then, after my tea, if there is still some noise, we will go down to the shelter."

She fell asleep and I went back to my bed, unhappy that I and the Soviet artillery could not make an impression on mother. I was thinking bitterly that her aloof elegance was inherited from her Polish princess mother, famous for utter nonchalance.

CSABA

Our academic education was designed to prepare us not only to ride but also to eventually teach and judge equitation. Therefore, we were also assigned pupils to mentor. I sharpened my pedagogic claws on a young man of about fourteen, who I will hide behind the invented name of Csaba. He had a sweet smile and very sad, outsized brown eyes, much like those made famous by the legendary poet, Endre Ady. The good news was that he possessed great talent for the equestrian arts. Beyond the elusive "riding talent" he possessed also the necessary character traits and the emotional and intellectual depth that must confluence with physical aptitude into the mighty flood of talent.

Around the 10th of November, Csaba telephoned me, as he frequently did. He was very disturbed and anxious about the traumatic events since the outbreak of the revolution on October 23rd. He actually lived in a battle zone, and for weeks he had been listening to gunfire. This morning he called to check if I was still alive. As he talked I could hear through the phone the enormous noises of war. He lived only a few buildings away from the famous Kilian Barracks, a courageous center of armed resistance against the Communist and Soviet forces, which was on the corner of Ulloi Avenue and Ferenc Boulevard. The garrisons of the Kilian Barracks were the first to mutineer from the Communist government and join the freedom fighters, giving them arms, ammunition and courage. Their brave leader was Colonel Pal Maleter, a disillusioned young Communist that turned on the Soviets to side with the causes of his compatriots.

The day was unusually mild and sunny. Csaba reluctantly confessed that he was very frightened of the perpetual fighting around him. Surely, Csaba also received the admonition of good upbringing, "Do not complain and do not explain." Only because of the incessant noises of gunfire would Csaba reluctantly complain. Even I felt as if I were under fire by what I could hear through the telephone. He said that he decided to dodge some bullets, walk out to the Tattersall and sleep there in the stables with the horses. He said that it was tranquil there and by now only the horses could calm him down. He asked if I would join him there. I declined.

The next morning, after the 6 AM curfew, I walked the great distance to the Tattersall to see my horses and make myself useful. When I arrived there I saw with horror the great damage an artillery barrage had inflicted on the central building of the riding school. There was rubble, silence and the sound of my boots on the cobblestones. A wounded stable boy came to me and told in stingy sentences what had happened.

Csaba had arrived and worked to help the diminished

118

stable staff. In the early afternoon he went to the main building of the Tattersall to take a shower. As he crossed the center of the building on his way to the shower, a Soviet tank pulled up to the outer gate of the riding school, turned to face the main building, aimed at the center door and fired. Csaba received the artillery barrage, which – in our language currency, "totaled him." Then, the tank pivoted with a "job well done," and rumbled away in the direction of Keleti railway terminal. Nobody could find any remains of the utterly vaporized Csaba, which heightened the tragedy. There were no remains of even fragments that could have been collected, and therefore there was no funeral. Csaba went to the horses to be safe, to have peace and tranquility, and I hope that where he arrived instead has given him all that he wished for. It was thus that my first devoted student perished.

THE OFFICERS

In competition officers rode in military uniforms and represented their riding club, "Honved." The most elegant, although not the most successful Honved competitor was a lieutenant I fictitiously name Pal Hollos. Slender, with perfect posture, chain-smoking, and with an infectiously cheerful disposition, he was universally liked. He reminded me of the "old world" officer types that always looked better on a ballroom floor than in battle and had a certain dash of a rascal in them. He was without edge or malice, genuine when congratulating all the riders who beat him in contest. Nothing but harmony, kindness and levity could come close to him.

By the beginning of November, the Soviet military commandant was confident that he would overpower the rising Hungarians with his newly arrived Soviet divisions and secure the country once again as a Soviet satellite. The Soviet commanders summoned the newly elevated General Maleter, who since October 29th had also been appointed Minister of Defense to discuss the terms of a cease-fire and the orderly withdrawal of Soviet forces from Budapest. General Maleter went to conference with the Soviet commandants at Tokol, near Budapest, on

November 3, 1956. As usual, and as anticipated by all of us who did not wear braces on our brains, the invitation was a ploy. Pal Maleter lead the delegation of a small entourage of trusted officers, among them Pal Hollos. That must have been the greatest distinction and honor to Lieutenant Hollos as by then General Maleter, deservedly, was venerated by the nation. During the conference in Tokol on the following day, November 4th, the entire Hungarian delegation of officers were, of course, arrested by the Soviets with utter disregard for international law.

I saw General Maleter only once, accidentally, but I hoped to be guided by fate to see him again. He was unforgettably handsome with a sculpted face, large, deep-set eyes of great intelligence and the expression of unbridled courage under up-sweeping eyebrows, accompanied by a smile of tranquility and wisdom. He was remarkably tall and his eyes searched faces as if he could see thoughts and feelings in others. He was considered a military genius, a disillusioned Communist and a hero for turning on the communist regime to fight for liberty. After the Soviets arrested him, he was imprisoned. He was given the usual grotesque "show trial" and was executed with Imre Nagy, the Prime Minister of free Hungary, on June 16th in 1958.

"Trust but verify," later suggested President Reagan. The execution of General Maleter verified, indeed, that one could not trust the Soviets.

Exactly twenty years later I met Colonel Maleter's sister, a baroness von Vecsey in Hollywood. She had a strong resemblance to the General and had married the Baron von Vecsey, an officer of the "old Hungarian army." They escaped from Hungary at the end of World War II to the safety of America. There she was widowed, raising her beautiful and interesting daughters. We reminisced about her famous brother at great emotional cost to the baroness. I enjoyed the glamorous Hollywood entourage of her daughters and am filled with gracious memories of those times.

CHAPTER 8

MEDITATION

"Nothing has really happened until it has been recorded." (Virginia Wolf). I wrote this book in reverence and in mourning for those thousands uselessly slaughtered by those ideologues that claim to "love humanity" while hating people. I hope that the dead rest better by knowing they did not die in vain; that someone still loves them.

During terrifying and trying years, horses let me escape into a meditative inner peace. They gave me relief from anxiety, unconditional friendship and affection. They gave me knowledge and a privileged life by allowing me participation in the equestrian arts. Horses, unexplainably, gave me a feeling of utter safety. I never felt threatened by them and the sense of apprehension preceding danger never visited me while riding. Horses were the sources of the many thrills young people crave. They helped me survive. I dedicated my equestrian career to paying back a deeply felt, large debt to them.

It is with gratitude that I remember my teachers, my grooms, my horses, wonderful friends and unsuccessful foes. After I escaped the horrors of Communism, I realized that I was the beneficiary of the finest equestrian education available to very few of my generation. My teachers understood their subject and could teach it. They were the vessels through whom the science and art of riding transmuted. They learned from the best schools and finest masters and became a priesthood loyal to horses and horsemanship. As all great knowledge tends to be, the equestrian knowledge my teachers handed me was intoxicating.

It was riding that sustained me in the darkest years of my life. In fact, daily riding made my life not only endurable, but also actually livable, even enjoyable.

Whoever discovered water was not a fish. When one lives in a totalitarian tyranny, with all its suffering, one is forced to accept fear as "normal." Of course, if one lives in constant terror for one's life, one forgets the sweetness of liberty and is forbidden the pursuit of happiness. The custodians of one's life and destiny are dangerous thugs, even if sometimes wearing suits and neckties, and may be secretly listening to American jazz recordings. Tyrannies make no secret that they own you. Terror is on full display; only strategic details are kept as great secrets. Everyone hauled away to prison, exile, forced labor or death was hauled between 1 and 4 AM, dragged from a sleep of exhaustion, jerked away from a loving family, under the cover of darkness.

The riding school was still an island meritocracy. Some riders were good, others great. In competition one could win and the others in the class did not, regardless of political party affiliation. Merit, achievement and fame still mattered in the performing arts and sports. However, nobody was indispensable and we all knew that. But there was a sense of serenity in our insane world. One could still do well and be actually rewarded for it.

I agree with the Ancient Greek philosophers that people consist of body, mind and soul, all of which need equal attention and cultivation to stay in harmonious balance. Riding horses for their edification and well-being nourished my spirit, satisfied my intellect and improved my body.

Beyond these considerations were the absolutely healing and life-sustaining effects riding had on me. When I rode, the world of cares, fears and hardships fell away. I found myself in a state of great emotional happiness and intellectual well-being. Isolated from the world, insulated from hurt and in unity with a very generous and gorgeous living being, all the worries seemed to have been lifted from me. Actually, when "I was deep in riding" as I phrased that state for myself, it felt as if I had awakened from a nightmare and found myself back in a sunny, rational, cheerful world of considerable beauty. In life "some trivia" happens to us but the rest of life is lived in the mind. Horses helped me not only to survive but also to have lived those years with happiness, optimism and good will.

And I got to America in one uninjured piece!

EPILOGUE

A TRIBUTE

In honor and respect for the equestrian tradition of which I was a beneficiary Hungarian Royal Riding and Driving Instructor Academy, Orkenytabor, Hungary. Hungary was part of the Austro-Hungarian Empire, ruled by Europe's oldest royal family, the Habsburgs. The thousand-year anniversary of the national existence of Hungary was celebrated in 1896 with the Imperial Couple, Emperor Francis Joseph and Empress Elizabeth, present in Budapest.

During the years of the so-called Dual Monarchy, from 1867 to 1918, Hungary's military was integrated into the Imperial army called, for short the "K. und K." Thorough and expert equestrian education was then done in military schools. Famous ones existed in the capitals of various member states and provinces of the imperial realm. The quintessential refinements of

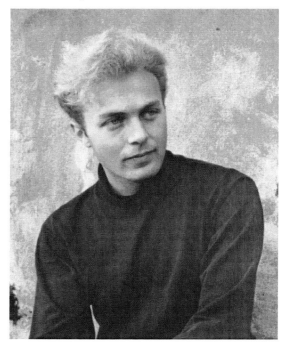

The author as under-graduate at the University of California, Berkeley.

correct equitation and the schooling of horses to the highest athletic achievements were done at the Imperial Spanish Riding School of

Vienna. Located in the very premises of the Viennese Imperial Palace, the school was founded in 1574 by the Emperor Charles V, and then maintained and patronized by the Imperial Family until the fall of the Habsburg Monarchy in 1918.

As a result of the First World War, the Austro-Hungarian Empire collapsed and according to the resolves of the Treaties of Versailles and Trianon, disintegrated. Its member parts became sovereign nation states, their boundaries often carelessly delineated, ignoring ethnic lines of demarcation. As a result of the Treaty of Trianon, only one third of the original territory of Hungary remained in Hungarian hands and became the Kingdom of Hungary.

After considerable civil unrest, foreign occupation and a brief insurrection of Communist terror, the nation was tranquilized under the rule of Admiral Miklos Horthy who was proclaimed the Regent of Hungary during the Inter-bellum years of 1920-44.

During the First World War the famous imperial riding schools, the Reitlehrerinstitute in Vienna and the Reit und Fahr Institute in Schlosshoff had closed their gates to further education of riding instructors. After the independence of the Hungarian Kingdom, the Hungarian Army established the Remount Training Team (Hungarian acronym P.I.K.) and housed it in the Franz Josef Barracks on the corner of Kerepesi Avenue and Hungaria Boulevard. Fated to become a famous equestrian educational institution, the P.I.K. was established on May 15, 1922. Its first Commandant was the Colonel Sandor Pronay.

The commandants and instructors of this prestigious institution were drawn from among the graduates of the Viennese Reitlehrerinstitute and were well-known and much respected riding masters from the times preceding the First World War. One of the greatest equestrian authorities of the time and an illustrious instructor at the defunct Viennese Reitlehrerinstitute, Colonel Zsigmond (Sigmund) Josipovich, emerged from retirement to insure that the P.I.K. would continue in Hungary with

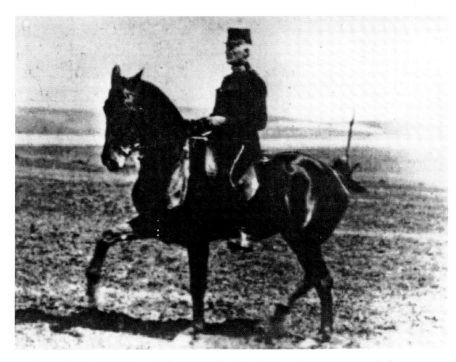

Colonel Zsigmond (Sigmund) Josipovich, emerged from retirement to insure that the PIK would continue in Hungary.

the great heritage of Classical Riding Art intact.

The flowering of the Hungarian riding art was a consequence of the successful blending of the campaign school [outdoor riding] of riding with the orthodoxy of the refinement of the schooled gaits and the devotion to collection on the haunches for balancing the traditional warhorse. This was the art advocating the natural horse moving in natural balance nimbly and with athletic strength rapidly through cross-country and over various obstacles, advocating the schooled horse's absolute obedience to the lightest of aids for the delivery of impeccably refined and educated natural movements of precision in outmost collection. The Hungarian National Riding Academy was in military hands and moved to its new home on Orkenytabor, about 50 miles Southeast of Budapest. The commissioned officers of the Royal Hungarian Army were selected from the members of the Hungarian nobility. They were also trained in classical horsemanship in the only Officers' School permitted to exist according to the terms of the disarmament, the famous Ludovica.

Adjacent to the royal palace in Budapest an imitation and sister institute to the Viennese Spanish Riding School was established in 1933. It, along with Orkenytabor and the Ludovica, were forced to close their doors by the Soviet occupation of 1945 and the following Communist Dictatorship. The very building that housed the Hungarian Spanish Riding School was destroyed by bombardment in 1944 and never rebuilt.

The advancing Soviet forces swept into Eastern Hungary in 1944 and completed their occupation of the country on April 9, 1945. Many officers of the Hungarian Royal Army retreated with their families from the approaching Soviet Red Army toward the territories likely to be occupied by British and American forces. Those who surrendered to the Western Allies eventually immigrated to the United States and Great Britain.

These officers were university educated and pursued careers mostly in engineering fields. Although they were excellently educated equestrians, few of them taught horseback riding in the United States for a career. Some of them became judges of dressage and jumping events. Many remained, however, in obscurity while others rose to equestrian prominence in their new home countries. Most of these educated horsemen from Hungary did serve as catalysts, bettering the riding and stimulating interest in American dressage. From the Second World War and through the sixties, dressage clientele had to be created by explaining the traditions and benefits of classical horsemanship. Those who did not make an effort to advocate dressage or jumping in the traditional manner did not create enough interest in their expertise.

Thus, a great body of Hungarian educated expertise remained untapped. Much knowledge remained dormant. Due to the harshness of immigration and personal traumas, these equestrians were glad to serve the sport when sought out. However, few of them made the effort to promote great career opportunities.

I quickly assembled the names of those that I knew were well-educated equestrians and known in the United States riding circles for their contributions. I will list 17 of them alphabetically:

Laddie Andahazi, Bela Buttykai, Agoston d'Endrody, de Demeter, Kalman von Jurenak, Bertalan de Nemethy, Janos de Kenyeres, C. de Reszke, Charles de Rethy, Dezso de Szilagyi, Andrew de Szinyai, Gabor Foltenyi, Konyot, Nandor Pauli-Hartman, Zoltan Stehlo, Charles Valko, and Jozsef Count Zichy.

Some of these names are well known because their owners contributed substantially to the international success of American riders. Others have written important books (d'Endrody, de Nemethy, de Szilagyi.) Their colleges and friends who remained stranded in Hungary taught me. I knew of many of them by scanning through the old St. Georg magazines and by listening to my teachers' anecdotes about them. Then, having come to the United States, I met most of them. I was aware of their great expertise and of the wealth of their knowledge and experience. I want to pay tribute to them and what they represent.

Hungary always prided itself as an "equestrian nation." The original Magyars occupied their current homeland as nomadic horsemen who came on horseback and while they settled into an agricultural society, continued to find horsemanship their dominating passion. In the national lore and in actuality, horsemanship loomed large in the Hungarian imagination as it had inspired, embellished and articulated its culture.

Hungarians love horses and respect equestrian expertise.